A Profile of
Health and Disease
in America

Obstetrics, Gynecology, and Infant Mortality

A Profile of
Health and Disease
in America

Obstetrics,
Gynecology,
and
Infant
Mortality

Wrynn Smith, Ph.D.

Facts On File Publications
New York, New York • Oxford, England

A Profile of Health and Disease in America: Obstetrics, Gynecology, and Infant Mortality

Copyright © 1987 by Wrynn Smith

Library of Congress Cataloging-in-Publication Data
Smith, Wrynn.

Obstetrics, gynecology, and infant mortality.

(A Profile of health and disease in America)
Bibliography: p.
Includes index.
1. Gynecology—United States—Statistics.
2. Obstetrics—United States—Statistics. 3. Infants—Mortality—Statistics. 4. United States—Statistics, Medical. I. Title. II. Series: Smith, Wrynn. Profile of health and disease in America. [DNLM: 1. Gynecology—United States—statistics. 2. Infant Mortality—United States. 3. Infant, Newborn, Diseases—occurrence—United States. 4. Obstetrics—United States—statistics. WA 900 AA1 S55]
RG106.4U6S65   1987   362.1'98'0973021   86-32838
ISBN 0-8160-1455-8

Series design: Jo Stein

Printed in the United States of America

10 9 8 7 6 5 4 3 2 1

CONTENTS

Preface

Just a few decades ago, treating the sick was a simple affair. The local family doctor, equipped with a small array of poultices and a sympathetic manner, did his best to fight disease. Knowledge, medicines, instrumentation, and surgical procedures developed slowly. Today, however, in the era of proliferating biotechnology, specialization, third-party financing, hospices, and surgicenters, medical school professors seem to relish telling their students that 50% of what they are learning will be obsolete five years after graduation.

The flow of information crossing the desk of busy health-care professionals trying to keep abreast of ever-accelerating developments in disease diagnosis, treatment, and prevention, as well as in the financing, organization, and delivery of health care, is often overwhelming. Clearly, the need to keep up is critical. To be informed, health-care professionals—be they practitioners, hospital administrators, health-care planners, policy makers, insurers, or hospital or pharmaceutical supply executives—must attend to material from many disconnected sources. These sources might include current editions of classic texts, weekly and monthly professional journals, current research papers presented at colloquia, and a steady stream of government bulletins and study publications from the Centers for Disease Control, NIH, the Center for Health Statistics, and foundation reports. As with the proverbial forest that can't be seen for the trees, the voluminous and fragmented form of this information often obscures the major changes and trends rapidly occurring in the health care field.

The task of a grant applicant to locate and collate statistical information when framing the need for his work is a research project in itself. The same is true of a researcher defining a hypothesis, a physician determining the current utilization of a particular therapy regimen or a hospital administrator projecting bed needs.

To help such workers and investigators, I decided to gather data from many sources into one comprehensive coordinated source, this series entitled *A Profile of Health and Disease in America*, that will serve as a handy and definitive resource tool for health professionals.

Each volume contains both historical and current statistics on the incidence, prevalence, and mortality of major diseases within one of the major medical specialties. I've presented data for different geographic areas within the United States as well as international data. I've also included information on the use of various medicines and surgical procedures. The length of a hospital stay, how it varies geographically or for patients based on sex, and treatment costs are included as are discussions of major controversies. Thus, the reader will easily find data on flu viruses, changes in virus strains, current fertility rates of American teenagers, changes in the obesity level of Americans, and the latest incidence of pertussis, with a discussion of the pros and cons of the pertussis vaccine and of how many men suffer from toxic shock syndrome. Those readers interested in digestive disease can find recent information from government surveys on problems as diverse as ulcers and hemorrhoids. The volume on mental disease provides a wealth of data on depressive symptomatology, drug usage, alcoholism, and homicide and puts the recent increase of teenage suicide in historical perspective.

Data sources include the 1983 Symposium on Cancer Treatment, Public Health Reports, the National Natality Survey; the NHANES Surveys; publications of the Atlanta Centers For Disease Control, and NIH publications, as well as those of the American Heart, Lung, and Blood Institute, The American Cancer Institute, and the Institute For Allergy and Infectious Disease. Published research articles are discussed and referenced, and each volume includes a bibliography that can be used by those seeking to go beyond initial review of pertinent health data. These comprehensive volumes on so many health topics need not be the last source consulted, but I think for those owning them they will always be the first.

Introduction

Demographers examining prehistoric skeletal remains estimate that the life expectancy of people in prehistoric times was 18 to 25 years. Many persons lived much longer, but so many died as infants, children, and adolescents that the average lifespan was short.

Evidence from Egyptian mummy remains and from Greek and Roman burial inscriptions reveal that people lived somewhat longer—between 25 and 30 years—in early historic times possibly with an increase of about 5 years in the late Roman period. But since such select records typically represent only upper class males, they probably indicate greater longevity than was likely for the average person in these societies.

Life expectancy did not increase from this time until the late 17th Century in Europe. Then, the estimated lifespan of the average man or woman was as high as 40 years. Prior to that time, gains were sporadic and often eradicated by recurrent plagues and famines. But by 1700, reasonably complete death records from England, France, Wales, and Scandinavia show the first recorded enduring decline in mortality rates.

One reason for this decline was the reduced incidence of widespread, devastating plagues. In the plague of 1348 to 1350, 25 million people died, and the population of Europe is estimated to have fallen by one-fourth. In 1720, the last major plague killed between one-third and three-fourths of the residents of Marseilles and other southern French cities. Although historians agree that the first major gains in survival can be correlated with a lower incidence of severe plague, there is no definitive consensus about why plagues abated or why the mortality rate in developed countries continued to fall beyond this first reduction.

Although some important advances in western medicine took place in the 18th Century, such as the introduction of smallpox vaccination, hospices and midwifery services, many commentators consider the major reason for decreasing mortality to be the general rise in living standards brought about by socioeconomic improvements.

Socioeconomic improvements included the development of better farm implements and fertilizers, crop rotation, and the introduction of corn from America, together with more efficient transportation for food distribution. All of these factors contributed to better nutrition and the end of famine in Europe after the Irish potato famine of 1840.

Another improvement in living standard was the increased use of soap for personal hygiene in England and Wales. It was followed by a drop in the incidence of intestinal-tract disease and diseases transmitted by body lice. A concommitant change in dress was the introduction of washable cotton underwear. Based on the suspicion that disease might arise from bad air, an emphasis was also placed on having more windows in houses for better ventilation.

Similar general improvements took place in public sanitation and sewage, while private sanitation improved with the invention of the water closet in 1778. Between 1840 and 1900, the average life expectancy of the northern European increased by 9 years to about 50 years of age. In the United States, it was 47.3 years.

During this period, fluctuating mortality rates were replaced by low stable ones. The change reflects the transition from an age of widespread pestilence and uncontrollable infectious disease that particularly affected the young, to one of less frequent and limited disease outbreaks. In our lifetime, death mainly strikes the old who suffer from degenerative diseases, and those with illness related to lifestyle and cultural factors such as a cholesterol-rich diet, smoking, and alcohol consumption.

By 1900, cardiovascular disease, a major degenerative disease, had become a leading cause of death. Only infectious diseases like influenza, tuberculosis, pneumonia, typhoid fever, and diptheria taken together surpassed it.

This volume reviews the major changes in life expectancy that have occurred in the United States and elsewhere since 1900. Two of the most dramatic changes have been the reduced mortality of the newborn and of women in childbirth. Medical developments in delivering babies, such as using forceps and perfecting the cesarean procedure have dramatically increased the survival rates of mother and child in the first crucial hours after delivery.

Similarly, modern "miracle" drugs, antibiotics, and vaccines have enabled new mothers, their older infants, and children to survive the ravages of infectious and epidemic diseases, such as bacterial pneumonia and smallpox, that otherwise would have killed them. Feared diseases such as diptheria, cholera, smallpox, typhoid fever, scarlatina, thrush, whooping cough, influenza, and pneumonia which had accounted for 50% of the total mortality in the United States in 1900 caused only 6% of all deaths by mid-century.

These statistics reflect substantial gains in postneonatal survival in developed nations. Although underdeveloped countries still struggle with disease and infection, particularly infant diarrheal infection, postneonatal survival in these countries has also risen thanks to worldwide programs to eliminate diseases such as smallpox, measles, and polio.

Even the poorest infants in industrialized nations, e.g., blacks and American Indians show striking gains in postneonatal survival. Yet, as of the eighties, the postneonatal period is still a more dangerous time for black infants than it is for white infants. Indeed, black infants are at a slightly greater risk of postneonatal death versus neonatal death than are white infants. During the first 28 days after birth, the black infant's chance of death is substantially higher than the white infant's due to conditions related to gestation and birth such as low birth weight.

The best news since the mid-1960s is the improvement in the neonatal condition and care of newborns. This change has markedly lowered neonatal mortality rates for both white and minority-group babies. Although neonatal health factors have been more difficult to modify than the environmental conditions affecting postneonatal survival, progress continues. Birth defects, either genetic or acquired during gestation, constitute a major cause of neonatal death and morbidity. Microsurgical techniques have greatly improved a baby's chance of surviving severe deformities such as heart irregularities. This is particularly welcome since data from the Birth Defects Monitoring Program of the Atlanta Center for Disease Control show that heart irregularities seem to be on the rise. Fortunately, other defects such as spina bifida, have been decreasing in incidence. Today, more is also known about the effects of a pregnant woman's exposure to agents such as the rubella virus, nicotine, and alcohol. These factors are correlated with low birth weight, maldevelopment, and birth defects.

Neonatal mortality has also been declining because of better prenatal care, more health education and certain cultural trends in fertility. The proportion of low birth weight infants has dropped since 1965, and low birth weight is the cause of 75% of all neonatal deaths. Fewer children are being born at low birth weights in the 1980s than in the 1950s mainly because women are bearing fewer children. High parity (the number of pregnancies a woman has) is positively related to low birth weight as is the close spacing of pregnancies and multiple pregnancies. In addition more perinatal intensive care units are equipped with state-of-the-art life-sustaining equipment and personnel trained in techniques that nurture the premature or low birth weight infant ($<$ 2500 g) help these immature babies survive.

Medical advances in detecting fetal genetic defects and fetal stress monitoring have made it possible to manage the health problems of fetuses and newborns in ways unimaginable just a decade ago. Likewise, modern delivery methods, including cesarean section, have helped lower the incidence of birth trauma.

Cesarean section has lowered maternal mortality as well. Today the procedure is much safer than it used to be. Still, this major operation is not totally without risk to mother and child. Alarm at its sudden increased use from 5% of all deliveries in 1969 to more than 15% in 1978 is prompting both investigation and admonition that it be reserved for mothers and infants at risk for vaginal delivery. The maternal mortality rate for cesarean delivery is still three times as high as for vaginal delivery. See Chapter 4 "Obstetrics," for a discussion of cesarean delivery.

This volume also furnishes current information on trends in abortion and contraception as well as on the performance rate of hysterectomies and tubal ligations. These data are gleaned from the Atlanta Centers for Disease Control and the National Survey on Family Growth. As new forms of birth control become popular and then fall into disfavor in the wake of side effect and injury revelations, the American woman and her spouse have modified their birth control practices.

The public and the medical community's sensitivity to news about a rise in hysterectomies in the 1970s is also evident in the reversal of this trend when it became apparent that without some reassessment one-half of all American women have had a hysterectomy.

Vigilant attention and quick response to new medical problems is reflected by toxic shock syndrome data. Similarly, delayed marriage and pregnancy, the rise in venereal disease rates, and the lack of adoptable children have focused attention on infertility. Many scientific strides have been made in helping infertile couples, who numbered over 6 million in the late 1970s and early-1980s, obtain wanted children.

A discussion of obstetric and gynecologic topics would be incomplete without reviewing the latest advances in embryo implantation, hormone stimulating therapy and surrogate motherhood (Chapter 5, "Gynecology"). Finally, discussion focuses on the everyday problems of female reproduction, from dysmenorrhea and menopause to endometriosis and pelvic inflammatory disease.

From the onset of menses through childbirth to menopause, female reproductive health and disease and neonatal mortality and morbidity are especially rewarding topics for discussion since gains in reproductive health have, more than any others, accounted for the great increase in life expectancy in this century as if, out of a desire to begin at the beginning, science and medicine have directed their first successful thrust against the primary and most pervasive assault on longevity facing humankind—being born.

Average Life Expectancy 1

I n 1900, the average life expectancy at birth in the United States was 46.6 years for white males and 48.7 for white females. The average lifespan for non-whites was 32.5 years for males and 33.5 for females. By 1980, this average expectancy was 70.7 for white males, 78.1 for white females, 63.8 for black males, and 72.5 for black females (Table 1–1).

Some people misunderstand the average life expectancy statistic to mean that most men and women in 1900 died at the age expressed in the statistic, e.g., that most white males died at age 46.6 years and that people in general did not live past mid-life. In fact, however, many people lived into their 60s, 70s, and beyond.

TRENDS IN AVERAGE LONGEVITY

The average life expectancy statistic reflects the average length of life when the age at death of all short-lived people (those who die in infancy and childhood) is added to the age at death of those who die in old age. In 1900, many more infant and child deaths had to be averaged with old-age deaths than in 1980. This is why the average lifespan at birth in 1900 was so much lower than it is today.

TABLE 1–1. Life Expectancy at Birth and at Age 65 Years, According to Race and Sex: United States, Selected Years 1900–1984 (Data are Based on the National Vital Statistics System)

SPECIFIED AGE AND YEAR	All Races			White			Black		
	Both sexes	Male	Female	Both sexes	Male	Female	Both sexes	Male	Female
At birth:	Remaining life expectancy in years								
1900[*][†]	47.3	46.3	48.3	47.6	46.6	48.7	33.0[‡]	32.5[‡]	33.5[‡]
1950[†]	68.2	65.6	71.1	69.1	66.5	72.2	60.7	58.9	62.7
1960[†]	69.7	66.6	73.1	70.6	67.4	74.1	63.2	60.7	65.9
1970	70.9	67.1	74.8	71.7	68.0	75.6	64.1	60.0	68.3
1971	71.1	67.4	75.0	72.0	68.3	75.8	64.6	60.5	68.9
1972	71.2	67.4	75.1	72.0	68.3	75.9	64.7	60.4	69.1
1973	71.4	67.6	75.3	72.2	68.5	76.1	65.0	60.9	69.3
1974	72.0	68.2	75.9	72.8	69.0	76.7	66.0	61.7	70.3
1975	72.6	68.8	76.6	73.4	69.5	77.3	66.8	62.4	71.3
1976	72.9	69.1	76.8	73.6	69.9	77.5	67.2	62.9	71.6
1977	73.3	69.5	77.2	74.0	70.2	77.9	67.7	63.4	72.0
1978	73.5	69.6	77.3	74.1	70.4	78.0	68.1	63.7	72.4
1979	73.9	70.0	77.8	74.6	70.8	78.4	68.5	64.0	72.9
1980	73.7	70.0	77.4	74.4	70.7	78.1	68.1	63.8	72.5
1981	74.2	70.4	77.8	74.8	71.1	78.4	68.9	64.5	73.2
1982	74.5	70.9	78.1	75.1	71.5	78.7	69.4	65.1	73.7
1983	74.6	71.0	78.1	75.2	71.7	78.7	69.6	65.4	73.6
1984[†][*]	74.7	71.1	78.3	75.3	71.8	78.8	69.7	65.5	73.7
At 65 Years:									
1900–1902[*][†]	11.9	11.5	12.2	—	11.5	12.2	—	10.4[‡]	11.4[‡]
1950[†]	13.9	12.8	15.0	—	12.8	15.1	13.9	12.9	14.9
1960[†]	14.3	12.8	15.8	14.4	12.9	15.9	13.9	12.7	15.1
1970	15.2	13.1	17.0	15.2	13.1	17.1	14.2	12.5	15.7
1971	15.2	13.2	17.1	15.3	13.2	17.2	14.3	12.7	15.8
1972	15.2	13.1	17.1	15.2	13.1	17.2	14.2	12.4	15.8
1973	15.3	13.2	17.2	15.4	13.2	17.3	14.1	12.5	15.7
1974	15.6	13.4	17.5	15.7	13.5	17.7	14.5	12.7	16.2
1975	16.1	13.8	18.1	16.1	13.8	18.2	15.0	13.1	16.7
1976	16.1	13.8	18.1	16.2	13.8	18.2	15.0	13.1	16.7
1977	16.4	14.0	18.4	16.5	14.0	18.5	15.2	13.3	16.9
1978	16.4	14.1	18.4	16.5	14.1	18.5	15.3	13.3	17.1
1979	16.7	14.3	18.7	16.8	14.4	18.8	15.5	13.5	17.3
1980	16.4	14.1	18.3	16.5	14.2	18.4	15.1	13.0	16.8
1981	16.7	14.3	18.6	16.7	14.4	18.7	15.5	13.4	17.3
1982	16.8	14.5	18.7	16.9	14.5	18.8	15.7	13.5	17.5
1983	16.7	14.5	18.6	16.8	14.5	18.7	15.5	13.4	17.3
1984[†][**]	16.8	14.5	18.7	16.9	14.6	18.8	15.6	13.4	17.5

*Death registration area only; the death registration area increased from 10 states and the District of Columbia in 1900 to the conterminous United States in 1933.
†Includes deaths of nonresidents of the United States.
‡Figure is for the all other population.
**Provisional data.

Sources: National Center for Health Statistics: *Vital Statistics Rates in the United States, 1940–1960*, by R. D. Grove and A. M. Hetzel. DHEW Pub. No. (PHS) 1677. Public Health Service, Washington. U.S. Government Printing Office, 1968; *Vital Statistics of the United States, 1970*, Vol. II, Mortality, Part A. DHEW Pub. No. (HRA) 75-1101. Health Resources Administration. Washington. U.S. Government Printing Office, 1974; Annual summary of births, deaths, marriages, and divorces, United States, 1984. *Monthly Vital Statistics Report*. Vol. 33-No. 13. DHHS Pub. No. (PHS) 84-1120. Public Health Service. Hyattsville, Md., Sept. 26, 1985; Unpublished data from the Division of Vital Statistics; Data computed by the Office of Research and Methodology from data compiled by the Division of Vital Statistics.

Table 1–1 underscores this point. The life expectancy of males and females, white and black, who survived to age 65 years in 1900 (having survived the dangerous early years of life when so many of their contemporaries died) was 76.9 years (65 + 11.9). The projected average number of years left for the 65-year-old in 1900 is greater than the span projected for infants born in 1984 (Table 1–1)!

Of course, when one compares 1984 infants to 1900 infants progress is evident in a 27.4 year-increase in lifespan. This reflects the greatly improved health and survival today of people in their earliest years. Similarly, a comparison of persons age 65 years in 1900 with those age 65 years in 1980 shows that their average lifespan has climbed from the 76.9 years mentioned earlier to 81.8 years. This improvement, although significant, is not nearly so impressive as the increase in lifespan for infants since 1900.

By the 1970s, other industrialized countries with similar life expectancy spans showed the same increased longevity. Some developed nations, such as Sweden, Switzerland, and Japan have higher average life expectancies than the United States (Table 1–2).

Table 1–3 shows the average U.S. life expectancy for males and females by race for specific ages from infancy through age 70 years. In 1900, the average life expectancy at birth showed an approximate 3-year advantage for females of all races. But by age 1 year, it fell to one of roughly 16 months. These data suggest that in 1900 male babies died at a much greater rate than female. Those males surviving to their first birthday had a life expectancy closer to their female contemporaries. At older ages from 20 to 70 years, the female advantage was just over 1 year.

By 1969 to 1971, the advantage at birth for white females over white males and black females over black males (the largest group encompassed by the "all other" designation) was 8 years, as the childbirth death rate for young women declined substantially from its early 1900s level. This edge persists for females until age 60 years when it then narrows to a 4-year difference for black females over black males. An approximate 8-year lifespan superiority of white females over white males narrows to 5 years. This is explained by the increase in heart disease among postmenopausal women.

As was seen in Table 1–1, the life expectancy of between 65.5 and 78.8 years for infants in 1978 is less than it is for the 85 year-old proven survivors who have lived through the life-threatening vicissitudes of infancy and later life. People this age in all racial and sex groups have an average remaining life expectancy of 90 or more years. Their age is averaged only with those who are older than they.

TABLE 1–2. Life Expectancy at Birth, According to Sex: Selected Countries, Selected Periods (Data are based on reporting by countries)

Country	Period	Life Expectancy (in years)	Period	Life Expectancy (in years)
Male:				
Japan	1976	72.2	1981	73.8
Sweden	1972–76	72.1	1981	73.1
Israel	1975	70.3	1981	72.7
Norway	1975–76	71.9	1980–81	72.5
Netherlands	1971–75	71.2	1980	72.4
Switzerland	1968–73	70.3	1977–78	72.0
Cuba	1970	68.5	1977–78	71.5
Australia	1965–67	67.6	1981	71.4
Denmark	1975–76	71.1	1980–81	71.1
Spain	1970	69.7	1975	70.4
England and Wales	1974–76	69.6	1978–80	70.4
Canada	1970–72	69.3	1975–77	70.2
Greece	1960–62	67.5	1970	70.1
France	1974	69.0	1978–80	70.1
United States	1975	68.7	1979	70.0
Federal Republic of Germany	1974–76	68.3	1979–81	69.9
Italy	1970–72	69.0	1974–77	69.7
Finland	1975	67.4	1981	69.5
New Zealand	1970–72	68.6	1975–77	69.0
Austria	1976	68.1	1980	69.0
German Democratic Republic	1969–70	68.9	1981	69.0
Singapore	1970	65.1	1980	68.9
Ireland	1970–72	68.8	1970–72	68.8
Bulgaria	1969–71	68.6	1974–76	68.7
Scotland	1971–73	67.2	1979–81	68.6
Female:				
Norway	1975–76	78.1	1980–81	79.2
Netherlands	1971–75	77.2	1980	79.2
Japan	1976	77.4	1981	79.1
Sweden	1972–76	77.8	1981	79.1
Switzerland	1968–73	76.2	1977–78	78.7
Australia	1965–67	74.2	1981	78.4
France	1974	76.9	1978–80	78.2
United States	1975	76.5	1979	77.8
Finland	1975	75.9	1981	77.8
Canada	1970–72	76.4	1975–77	77.5
Denmark	1975–76	76.8	1980–81	77.2
Federal Republic of Germany	1974–76	74.8	1979–81	76.7
England and Wales	1974–76	75.8	1978–80	76.6
Spain	1970	75.0	1975	76.2
Austria	1976	75.1	1980	76.2
Italy	1970–72	74.9	1974–77	75.9
Isreal	1975	73.9	1981	75.9
New Zealand	1970–72	74.6	1975–77	75.5
Poland	1976	74.6	1981	75.2
Belgium	1968–72	74.2	1972–76	75.1
Cuba	1970	71.8	1977–78	74.9
Scotland	1971–73	73.6	1979–81	74.9

TABLE 1–2. (Continued)

Country	Period	Life Expectancy (in years)	Period	Life Expectancy (in years)
German Democratic Republic	1969–70	74.2	1981	74.8
Czechoslovakia	1977	73.6	1981	74.3
Singapore	1970	70.0	1980	74.2

Note: Rankings are from highest to lowest life expectancy based on the latest available data for countries or geographic areas with at least 1 million population and most recent data for 1970 or later. This table is based only on data from the official life tables of the country concerned, consistent with the data in the United Nations *Demographic Yearbook, 1982*.

Sources: United Nations: *Demographic Yearbook, 1977* and *1982*. Pub. Nos. ST/ESA/STAT/SER.R/6 and ST/ESA/STAT/SER.R/12. New York. United Nations, 1978 and 1984; National Center for Health Statistics: Unpublished data from the Division of Vital Statistics.

TABLE 1–3. Life Table Values by Color, Age, and Sex for United States 1900–1978

AGE, COLOR, AND SEX	Average number of years of life remaining								
	1978*	1969–71*	1959–61	1949–51	1939–41	1929–31	1919–21	1909–11	1900–02
White Male:									
0	70.2	67.94	67.55	66.31	62.81	59.12	56.34	50.23	48.23
1	70.1	68.33	68.34	67.41	64.98	62.04	60.24	56.26	54.61
5	66.3	64.55	64.61	63.77	61.68	59.38	58.31	55.37	54.43
10	61.5	59.69	59.78	58.98	57.03	54.96	54.15	51.32	50.59
15	56.6	54.83	54.93	54.18	52.33	50.39	49.74	46.91	46.25
20	52.0	50.22	50.25	49.52	47.76	46.02	45.60	42.71	42.19
25	47.5	45.70	45.65	44.93	43.28	41.78	41.60	38.79	38.52
30	42.8	41.07	40.97	40.29	38.80	37.54	37.65	34.87	34.88
35	38.2	36.43	36.31	35.68	34.36	33.33	33.74	31.08	31.29
40	33.6	31.87	31.73	31.17	30.03	29.22	29.86	27.43	27.74
45	29.1	27.48	27.34	26.87	25.87	25.28	26.00	23.86	24.21
50	24.8	23.34	23.22	22.83	21.96	21.51	22.22	20.39	20.76
55	20.8	19.51	19.45	19.11	18.34	17.97	18.59	17.03	17.42
60	17.2	16.07	16.01	15.76	15.05	14.72	15.25	13.98	14.35
65	14.0	13.02	12.97	12.75	12.07	11.77	12.21	11.25	11.51
70	11.1	10.38	10.29	10.07	9.42	9.20	9.51	8.83	9.03
75	8.6	8.06	7.92	7.77	7.17	7.02	7.30	6.75	6.84
80	6.7	6.18	5.89	5.88	5.38	5.26	5.47	5.09	5.10
85	5.3	4.63	4.34	4.35	4.02	3.99	4.06	3.88	3.81
All Other Male:									
0	65.0	60.98	61.48	58.91	52.33	47.55	47.14	34.05	32.54
1	65.5	62.13	63.50	61.06	56.05	51.08	51.63	42.53	42.46
5	61.8	58.48	59.98	57.69	53.13	48.69	50.18	44.25	45.06
10	57.0	53.67	55.19	52.96	48.54	44.27	45.99	40.65	41.90
15	52.1	48.84	50.39	48.23	43.95	39.83	41.75	36.77	38.26
20	47.4	44.37	45.78	43.73	39.74	35.95	38.38	33.46	35.11
25	43.1	40.29	41.38	39.49	35.94	32.67	35.54	30.44	32.21
30	38.8	36.20	37.05	35.31	32.25	29.45	32.51	27.33	29.25
35	34.5	32.16	32.81	31.21	28.67	26.39	29.54	24.42	26.18
40	30.4	28.29	28.72	27.29	25.23	23.36	26.53	21.57	23.12
45	26.5	24.64	24.89	23.59	22.02	20.59	23.55	18.85	20.09
50	22.8	21.24	21.28	20.25	19.18	17.92	20.47	16.21	17.34
55	19.5	18.14	18.11	17.36	16.67	15.46	17.50	13.82	14.69
60	16.5	15.35	15.29	14.91	14.38	13.15	14.74	11.67	12.62
65	14.1	12.87	12.84	12.75	12.18	10.87	12.07	9.74	10.38
70	11.6	10.68	10.81	10.74	10.06	8.78	9.58	8.00	8.33

TABLE 1-3. (Continued)

AGE, COLOR, AND SEX	Average number of years of life remaining								
	1978*	1969–71*	1959–61	1949–51	1939–41	1929–31	1919–21	1909–11	1900–02
All Other Male:									
75	9.8	8.99	8.93	8.83	8.09	6.99	7.61	6.58	6.60
80	8.8	7.57	6.87	7.07	6.46	5.42	5.83	5.53	5.12
85	7.8	6.04	5.08	5.38	5.08	4.30	4.53	4.48	4.04
White Female:									
0	77.8	75.49	74.19	72.03	67.29	62.67	58.53	53.62	51.08
1	77.6	75.66	74.68	72.77	68.93	64.93	61.51	58.69	56.39
5	73.8	71.86	70.92	69.09	65.57	62.17	59.43	57.67	56.03
10	68.9	66.97	66.05	64.26	60.85	57.65	55.17	53.57	52.15
15	64.0	62.07	61.15	59.39	56.07	53.00	50.67	49.12	47.79
20	59.1	57.24	56.29	54.56	51.38	48.52	46.46	44.88	43.77
25	54.3	52.42	51.45	49.77	46.78	44.25	42.55	40.88	40.05
30	49.5	47.60	46.63	45.00	42.21	39.99	38.72	36.96	36.42
35	44.6	42.82	41.84	40.28	37.70	35.73	34.88	33.09	32.82
40	39.9	38.12	37.13	35.64	33.25	31.52	30.94	29.26	29.17
45	35.2	33.54	32.53	31.12	28.90	27.39	26.98	25.45	25.51
50	30.7	29.11	28.08	26.76	24.72	23.41	23.12	21.74	21.89
55	26.4	24.85	23.81	22.58	20.73	19.60	19.40	18.18	18.43
60	22.3	20.79	19.69	18.64	17.00	18.05	15.93	14.92	15.23
65	18.4	16.93	15.88	15.00	13.56	12.81	12.75	11.97	12.23
70	14.8	13.37	12.38	11.68	10.50	9.98	9.94	9.38	9.59
75	11.5	10.21	9.28	8.87	7.92	7.56	7.62	7.20	7.33
80	8.8	7.59	6.67	6.59	5.88	5.63	5.70	5.35	5.50
85	6.7	5.54	4.66	4.83	4.34	4.24	4.24	4.06	4.10
All Other Female:									
0	73.6	69.05	66.47	62.70	55.51	49.51	46.92	37.67	35.04
1	74.0	70.01	68.10	64.37	58.47	52.33	50.39	45.15	43.54
5	70.2	66.34	64.54	60.93	55.47	49.81	48.70	48.42	46.04
10	65.4	61.49	59.72	56.17	50.83	45.33	44.54	42.84	43.02
15	60.4	56.60	54.85	51.36	46.22	40.87	40.36	39.18	39.79
20	55.6	51.85	50.07	46.77	42.14	37.22	37.15	36.14	38.89
25	50.9	47.19	45.40	42.35	38.31	33.93	34.35	32.97	33.90
30	46.2	42.61	40.83	38.02	34.52	30.67	31.48	29.61	30.70
35	41.5	38.14	36.41	33.82	30.83	27.47	28.58	26.44	27.52
40	37.0	33.87	32.16	29.82	27.31	24.30	25.60	23.34	24.37
45	32.7	29.80	29.14	26.07	24.00	21.39	22.61	20.43	21.36
50	28.5	25.97	24.31	22.67	21.04	18.60	19.76	17.65	18.67
55	24.7	22.37	20.89	19.62	18.44	16.27	17.09	14.98	15.88
60	21.2	19.02	17.83	16.95	16.14	14.22	14.69	12.78	13.60
65	18.0	15.99	15.12	14.54	13.95	12.24	12.41	10.82	11.38
70	14.8	13.30	12.46	12.29	11.91	10.38	10.25	9.22	9.62
75	12.5	11.06	10.10	10.15	9.80	8.62	8.37	7.55	7.90
80	11.5	9.01	7.66	8.15	8.00	6.90	6.58	6.05	6.48
85	9.9	7.07	5.44	6.15	6.38	5.48	5.22	5.09	5.10

*Deaths of nonresidents of the United States were excluded beginning in 1970.
Source: *Vital Statistics of the U.S., Natality* Vol. 1, 1978

DEATH RATES

A steady decline in both the crude death rate (the number of deaths per 100,000 general population) and age-adjusted death rate (number of deaths per 100,000 corrected for population changes in high mortality risk age groups that could mask a true rate) is shown in Fig. 1–1 for the United States since the 1930s.

While the overall U.S. mortality rate has been declining in this century, the rates for different sex and racial cohorts have varied considerably. The mortality rate by sex and race since 1900 is shown in Table 1–4. Both non-white men and women historically have had a higher mortality rate than white men and women. Similarly, women in 1900 had a slightly lower mortality than men of the same race. This difference between the sexes of both races has grown substantially since the turn of the century with the advent of medical advances in both maternal care and infant delivery.

A lower death rate for women than men by race in every age category from infancy through 85 years of age can be seen in Table 1–5. But the death rate for black females age under 1 year in 1984 at 1841.3 per 100,000, although lower than that for black males at 2,221.8, was still higher than that for white males at 997.4 per 100,000. Not until age 5 to 14 years do black females, like white females have a lower death rate than white males. A shift in the 5-to-14-year-old category whereby black females show a lower death rate than white males is first seen in 1970 (Table 1–5).

One can also see a racial mortality "crossover" referred to by several scholars, such as Manton[a] (Table 1–5). The crossover occurs when the death rate of non-whites becomes lower than that for whites in advanced age categories.

White males age 85 years and older in 1984 had a death rate of 18,511.5 per 100,000, whereas black males in the same age bracket had a rate of only 14,707.7 per 100,000 (Table 1–5). Until 1970, this crossover could be seen at ages 75 to 84 years as well. But by 1980, the differential in rates had reverted to the usual pattern of a higher mortality rate for blacks than for whites. In explanation of this phenomenon, researchers believe that the higher mortality for minorities at early ages leaves only the strongest surviving to advanced age.

Although data for other minorities are scarce, researchers found a similar crossover effect studying the Spanish surname popula-

---

[a]Manton KG: Sex and race specific differentials in multiple cause of death data. *Gerontologist* 20: 480–493, 1980

FIG. 1–1.   Crude and age-adjusted death rates: 1930–82

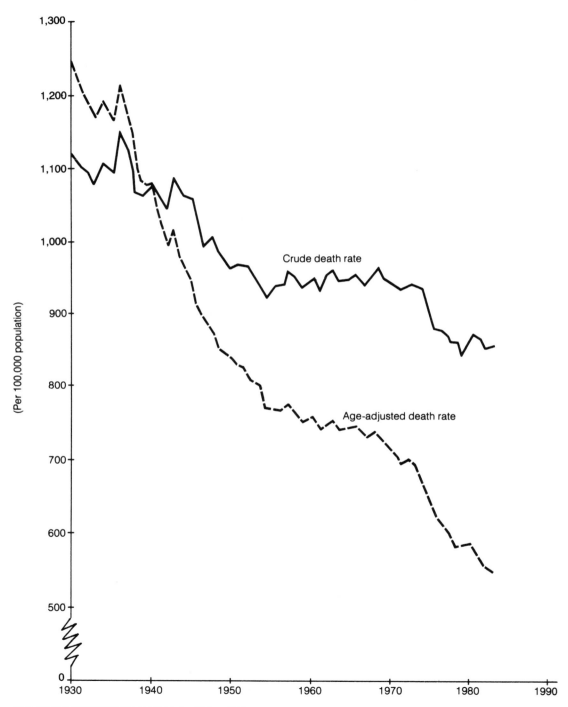

TABLE 1–4. Age-Adjusted Death Rates by Color and Sex: Death-Registration States, 1900–1932, and United States, 1933–78, 1983, (Rates per 1,000 population. Computed by the direct method, using as the standard population the age distribution of the total population of the United States as enumerated in 1940)

Area and Year	Total			White			All Other		
	Both sexes	Male	Female	Both sexes	Male	Female	Both sexes	Male	Female
United States:									
1983	5.5								
1982	6.6								
1978*	6.1	8.0	4.5	5.8	7.7	4.3	8.0	10.3	6.1
1977*	6.1	8.1	4.5	5.9	7.8	4.3	8.1	10.5	6.2
1976*	6.3	8.3	4.6	6.0	8.0	4.4	8.3	10.7	6.4
1975*	6.4	8.5	4.7	6.1	8.1	4.5	8.5	11.0	6.5
1974*	6.7	8.8	4.9	6.4	8.4	4.7	9.0	11.5	6.9
1973*	6.9	9.1	5.1	6.6	8.7	4.8	9.5	12.1	7.4
1972*,†	7.0	9.2	5.2	6.7	8.8	4.9	9.7	12.3	7.5
1971*	7.0	9.2	5.2	6.7	8.8	4.9	9.6	12.1	7.5
1970*	7.1	9.3	5.3	6.8	8.9	5.0	9.8	12.3	7.7
1969	7.3	9.5	5.4	6.9	9.1	5.1	10.2	12.7	8.0
1968	7.4	9.7	5.6	7.1	9.2	5.2	10.5	12.9	8.3
1967	7.3	9.4	5.5	6.9	9.0	5.1	9.9	12.1	8.0
1966	7.4	9.5	5.6	7.1	9.2	5.3	10.2	12.4	8.3
1965	7.4	9.5	5.6	7.0	9.1	5.3	10.1	12.2	8.3
1964	7.4	9.4	5.7	7.1	9.1	5.3	10.2	12.1	8.5
1963‡	7.6	9.6	5.8	7.2	9.2	5.4	10.5	12.4	8.8
1962‡	7.5	9.4	5.8	7.1	9.0	5.4	10.2	11.9	8.7
1961	7.4	9.2	5.7	7.0	8.9	5.4	10.0	11.6	8.5
1960	7.6	9.5	5.9	7.3	9.2	5.6	10.5	12.1	8.9
1959	7.5	9.3	5.9	7.2	9.0	5.5	10.3	11.9	8.8
1958	7.6	9.4	6.0	7.3	9.1	5.6	10.6	12.2	9.2
1957	7.8	9.6	6.1	7.4	9.2	5.7	10.8	12.4	9.4
1956	7.6	9.4	6.0	7.3	9.1	5.7	10.5	11.9	9.1
1955	7.6	9.3	6.1	7.3	9.1	5.7	10.4	11.9	9.1
1954	7.6	9.3	6.1	7.3	9.0	5.7	10.6	12.0	9.2
1953	8.0	9.8	6.4	7.7	9.4	6.1	11.4	13.0	9.9
1952	8.2	9.8	6.6	7.8	9.4	6.2	11.7	13.3	10.2
1951	8.3	9.9	6.7	7.9	9.6	6.3	11.9	13.3	10.5
1950	8.4	10.0	6.9	8.0	9.6	6.5	12.3	13.6	11.0
1949	8.5	10.1	7.0	8.1	9.7	6.6	12.3	13.5	11.1
1948	8.8	10.3	7.3	8.3	10.0	6.8	12.5	13.8	11.2
1947	9.0	10.5	7.5	8.6	10.1	7.1	12.5	13.6	11.4
1946	9.1	10.6	7.7	8.8	10.2	7.3	12.4	13.5	11.3
1945	9.5	11.1	8.0	9.1	10.7	7.5	13.1	14.5	11.9
1944	9.7	11.2	8.3	9.3	10.8	7.8	13.8	14.9	12.6
1943	10.2	11.6	8.7	9.7	11.2	8.2	14.5	15.7	13.4
1942	9.9	11.4	8.5	9.4	10.9	8.0	14.5	15.8	13.3
1941	10.3	11.7	8.9	9.7	11.2	8.3	15.6	16.9	14.3
1940	10.8	12.1	9.4	10.2	11.6	8.8	16.3	17.6	15.0
1939	10.7	12.0	9.5	10.2	11.4	8.9	16.0	17.1	14.9
1938	10.9	12.1	9.7	10.3	11.5	9.1	16.6	17.7	15.5

TABLE 1–4. (Continued)

Area and Year	Total Both sexes	Total Male	Total Female	White Both sexes	White Male	White Female	All Other Both sexes	All Other Male	All Other Female
United States:									
1937	11.7	13.1	10.3	11.1	12.4	9.7	17.8	19.2	16.3
1936	12.2	13.5	10.8	11.5	12.8	10.1	18.5	20.1	17.0
1935	11.6	12.9	10.4	11.1	12.3	9.8	17.3	18.5	16.1
1934	11.9	13.1	10.7	11.3	12.5	10.0	17.9	19.0	16.7
1933	11.6	12.7	10.5	11.0	12.2	9.9	17.2	18.1	16.4
Death-Registration States*									
1932	11.9	12.9	10.8	11.3	12.3	10.2	17.8	18.6	17.0
1931	12.1	13.2	11.0	11.4	12.5	10.3	19.0	19.9	18.1
1930	12.5	13.5	11.3	11.7	12.8	10.6	20.1	21.0	19.2
1929	13.2	14.2	12.1	12.4	13.5	11.4	21.0	21.9	20.0
1928	13.4	14.4	12.3	12.6	13.6	11.5	20.9	21.7	20.2
1927	12.6	13.5	11.6	11.9	12.8	10.9	19.8	20.4	19.3
1926	13.5	14.3	12.5	12.7	13.6	11.8	21.4	22.1	20.8
1925	13.0	13.8	12.2	12.3	13.2	11.4	20.9	21.4	20.4
1924	12.9	13.7	12.1	12.2	13.1	11.3	20.5	21.1	20.0
1923	13.5	14.2	12.8	12.9	13.7	12.1	19.8	20.0	19.7
1922	13.0	13.7	12.4	12.6	13.3	11.8	18.3	18.4	18.4
1921	12.7	13.2	12.1	12.2	12.7	11.6	18.2	18.0	18.6
1920	14.2	14.7	13.8	13.7	14.2	13.1	20.6	20.4	21.0
1919	14.0	14.6	13.4	13.4	14.1	12.8	20.5	20.3	20.8
1918	19.0	20.9	17.3	18.4	20.2	16.6	28.0	28.9	27.1
1917	15.3	16.5	14.0	14.7	16.0	13.4	23.4	24.1	22.7
1916	15.1	16.2	13.9	14.7	15.8	13.4	22.2	22.6	21.6
1915	14.4	15.4	13.4	14.1	15.1	13.0	23.1	23.5	22.6
1914	14.5	15.6	13.4	14.1	15.2	13.0	22.6	23.3	21.9
1913	15.0	16.1	13.7	14.6	15.8	13.4	22.7	23.3	22.0
1912	14.8	16.0	13.7	14.6	15.7	13.4	23.1	24.0	22.2
1911	15.2	16.2	14.1	14.9	15.9	13.8	23.7	24.4	22.9
1910	15.8	16.9	14.6	15.6	16.7	14.4	24.1	24.8	23.2
1909	15.3	16.3	14.2	15.0	16.1	14.0	24.1	24.8	23.3
1908	15.8	16.8	14.6	15.5	16.6	14.4	24.7	25.3	24.1
1907	17.1	18.4	15.7	16.8	18.2	15.4	26.6	27.5	25.7
1906	16.7	17.9	15.4	16.4	17.6	15.1	26.2	27.0	25.5
1905	16.7	17.8	15.7	16.5	17.6	15.4	28.3	29.7	26.9
1904	17.3	18.4	16.2	17.1	18.1	16.0	29.1	30.7	27.4
1903	16.5	17.4	15.5	16.2	17.2	15.3	27.2	28.5	25.9
1902	16.2	17.2	15.1	16.0	17.0	14.9	25.9	27.5	24.5
1901	17.2	18.2	16.2	17.0	18.0	16.0	26.9	28.4	25.5
1900	17.8	18.6	17.0	17.6	18.4	16.8	27.8	28.7	27.1

*Excludes deaths of nonresidents of the United States.
†Deaths based on a 50-percent sample.
‡Figures by color exclude data for residents of New Jersey.
**Increased in number from 10 States and the District of Columbia in 1900 to the entire conterminous United States in 1933.
Source: *Colonial Statistics of the United States*

TABLE 1–5.   Death Rates for All Causes, According to Sex, Race, and Age: United States, Selected Years 1950–84 (Data are based on the National Vital Statistics System)

SEX, RACE, AND AGE (IN YEARS)	1950*	1960*	1970	1980	1981	1982	1983	1984*,†
All Races:	Number of deaths per 100,000 resident population							
All ages, age-adjusted	841.5	760.9	714.3	585.8	568.2	553.8	550.5	547.7
All ages, crude	963.8	954.7	945.3	878.3	862.4	852.0	862.8	866.8
Under 1	3,299.2	2,696.4	2,142.4	1,288.3	1,207.3	1,164.2	1,107.3	1.077.8
1–4	139.4	109.1	84.5	63.9	60.2	57.6	55.9	50.1
5–14	60.1	46.6	41.3	30.6	29.4	28.3	26.9	25.1
15–24	128.1	106.3	127.7	115.4	107.1	101.0	96.0	98.5
25–34	178.7	146.4	157.4	135.5	132.1	125.2	121.4	123.1
35–44	358.7	299.4	314.5	227.9	221.3	207.4	201.9	205.5
45–54	853.9	756.0	730.0	584.0	573.5	549.7	535.7	531.7
55–64	1,911.7	1,735.1	1,658.8	1,346.3	1,322.1	1,297.9	1,299.5	1,289.6
65–74	4,067.7	3,822.1	3,582.7	2,994.9	2,922.3	2,885.2	2,874.3	2,864.4
75–84	9,331.1	8,745.2	8,004.4	6,692.6	6,429.9	6,329.8	6,441.5	6,416.5
85 and over	20,196.9	19,857.5	17,539.4	15,980.3	15,379.7	15,048.3	15,168.0	14,890.1
White Male:								
All ages, age-adjusted	963.1	917.7	893.4	745.3	724.4	706.0	698.4	694.6
All ages, crude	1,089.5	1,098.5	1,086.7	983.3	965.1	951.8	957.4	961.8
Under 1	3,400.5	2,694.1	2,113.2	1,230.3	1,182.0	1,135.5	1,052.9	997.4
1–4	135.5	104.9	83.6	66.1	60.5	58.2	57.3	52.1
5–14	67.2	52.7	48.0	35.0	34.2	32.5	31.1	28.4
15–24	152.4	143.7	170.8	167.0	154.5	145.6	137.0	141.9
25–34	185.3	163.2	176.6	171.3	167.3	158.7	154.8	160.5
35–44	380.9	332.6	343.5	257.4	252.4	238.6	232.9	234.2
45–54	984.5	932.2	882.9	698.9	686.5	659.9	636.5	633.4
55–64	2,304.4	2,225.2	2,202.6	1,728.5	1,692.0	1,654.6	1,642.9	1,622.3
65–74	4,864.9	4,848.4	4,810.1	4,035.7	3,926.9	3,859.8	3,816.1	3,783.4
75–84	10,526.3	10,299.6	10,098.8	8,829.8	8,565.2	8,444.7	8,556.9	8,511.2
85 and over	22,116.3	21,750.0	20,392.6	19,097.3	18,454.0	18,123.1	18,443.3	18,511.5
Black Male:								
All ages, age-adjusted	1,373.1	1,246.1	1,318.6	1,112.8	1,067.7	1,035.0	1,019.6	1,016.1
All ages, crude	1,260.3	1,181.7	1,186.6	1,034.1	991.6	960.4	963.3	963.4
Under 1	1,412.6	5,306.8	4,298.9	2,586.7	2,164.8	2,168.9	2,243.4	2,221.8
1–4		208.5	150.5	110.5	105.3	93.4	96.8	84.2
5–14	95.1	75.1	67.1	47.4	45.2	44.4	40.9	43.7
15–24	289.7	212.0	320.6	209.1	186.7	175.4	165.0	163.2
25–34	503.5	402.5	559.5	407.3	387.1	360.3	335.8	329.2
35–44	878.1	762.0	956.6	689.8	667.9	606.7	586.5	608.9
45–54	1,905.0	1,624.8	1,777.5	1,479.9	1,432.5	1,352.1	1,287.3	1,291.1
55–64	3,773.2	3,316.4	3,256.9	2,873.0	2,804.1	2,758.1	2,713.1	2,656.6
65–74	5,310.3	5,798.7	5,803.2	5,131.1	5,046.3	5,040.1	4,949.3	4,991.7
75–84	10,101.9	8,605.1	9,454.9	9,231.6	8,635.1	8,477.2	9,100.0	8,869.0
85 and over		14,844.8	14,415.4	16,098.8	15,396.4	15,117.9	14,155.6	14,707.7
White Female:								
All ages, age-adjusted	645.0	555.0	501.7	411.1	401.4	393.3	392.7	391.4
All ages, crude	803.3	800.9	812.6	806.1	799.6	797.9	815.3	822.1
Under 1	2,566.8	2,007.7	1,614.6	962.5	935.4	895.2	837.6	826.5
1–4	112.2	85.2	66.1	49.3	47.7	47.0	43.9	39.4

TABLE 1–5. (Continued)

SEX, RACE, AND AGE (IN YEARS)	1950*	1960*	1970	1980	1981	1982	1983	1984*,†
White Female:								
5–14	45.1	34.7	29.9	22.9	21.6	21.2	19.7	18.6
15–24	71.5	54.9	61.6	55.5	53.2	49.5	48.3	50.1
25–34	112.8	85.0	84.1	65.4	64.7	61.3	60.1	58.4
35–44	235.8	191.1	193.3	138.2	133.6	127.7	123.4	123.4
45–54	546.4	458.8	462.9	372.7	370.9	355.1	351.0	351.6
55–64	1,293.8	1,078.9	1,014.9	876.2	869.4	859.8	867.8	866.6
65–74	3,242.8	2,779.3	2,470.7	2,066.6	2,032.8	2,022.9	2,024.7	2,031.4
75–84	8,481.5	7,696.6	6,698.7	5,401.7	5,176.3	5,100.7	5,162.2	5,161.7
85 and over	19,679.5	19,477.7	16,729.5	14,979.6	14,438.2	14,123.9	14,278.3	13,909.5
Black Female:								
All ages, age-adjusted	1,106.7	916.9	814.4	631.1	599.1	581.4	590.4	586.2
All ages, crude	1,002.0	905.0	829.2	733.3	707.3	692.4	711.2	711.1
Under 1 ⎫	1,139.3	4,162.2	3,368.8	2,123.7	1,823.4	1,760.1	1,818.6	1,841.3
1–4 ⎬		173.3	129.4	84.4	81.6	76.4	73.6	68.3
5–14 ⎭	72.8	53.8	43.8	30.5	30.0	29.4	28.0	24.5
15–24	213.1	107.5	111.9	70.5	64.0	63.5	65.6	69.1
25–34	393.3	273.2	231.0	150.0	141.1	134.8	130.0	129.7
35–44	758.1	568.5	533.0	323.9	306.1	282.7	276.1	309.3
45–54	1,576.4	1,177.0	1,043.9	768.2	723.9	693.1	685.8	641.0
55–64	3,089.4	2,510.9	1,986.2	1,561.0	1,527.9	1,498.3	1,526.3	1,525.6
65–74	4,000.2	4,064.2	3,860.9	3,057.4	2,929.7	2,863.0	2,930.6	2,881.7
75–84 ⎫	8,347.0	6,730.0	6,691.5	6,212.1	5,822.3	5,708.5	6,064.6	6,095.1
85 and over ⎭		13,052.6	12,131.7	12,367.2	11,933.0	11,660.0	11,329.5	10,729.9

*Includes deaths of nonresidents of the United States
†Provisional data
Sources: National Center for Health Statistics: *Vital Statistics of the United States,* Vol. II, Mortality, Part A, 1950–83. Public Health Service. Washington. U.S. Government Printing Office; Annual summary of births, deaths, marriages, and divorces, United States, 1984. *Monthly Vital Statistics Report.* Vol. 33-No. 13. DHHS Pub. No. (PHS) 84-1120. Public Health Service. Hyattsville, Md., Sept. 26, 1985; Data computed by the Division of Analysis from data compiled by the Division of Vital Statistics

tion in Texas. Life expectancy among Spanish surname males was much higher than that of blacks and was similar to that of the white majority population until age 65 years. At that age, Spanish males actually showed a greater life expectancy than did white males.

Carr and Lee studying the American Indian population in the mid-1970s did not find a crossover effect for this group. The mortality profile among the Navajo population differed markedly from other American groups in that the major cause of death was accident, particularly motor vehicle accident.[b]

The Indian male life expectancy at birth was only 58.8 years compared to 71.8 years for Indian females. Navajo women had a

---

[b]Kyriakos S. Markides: Mortality among minority populations: a review of recent patterns and trends. *Public Health Reports* 98: 252–260, May–June 1983

profile closer to that of other American groups except that the second leading cause of death for them was accidental death. The leading cause of death among Indian women was ischemic heart disease, just as it is for the general population.

DEATH RATES BY MAJOR CAUSE

The great leap in average longevity at birth in the United States from about 40 years in 1900 for all segments of the population to an average of over 70 years in 1983 can be attributed to pharmaceutical advances. Drugs like penicillin and other antibiotics have been effective against several forms of pneumonia, syphilis, gangrene, rheumatic fever, cholera, sepsis, and staphylococcal infections. Antitubercular drugs have been used not only for treatment but prophylactically. Tuberculosis has also become rare, because of widespread screening of the population to detect and control it and recovery sanitaria.

Other infectious diseases, including polio, smallpox, diptheria, whooping cough, and many childhood diseases, such as measles and mumps have been prevented by inoculation. This measure is often mandated by law and provided free by public health authorities. United States public health contributions to greater longevity include the chlorination of water supplies in 1908, the pasteurization of milk in 1909, and improvements in personal hygiene and private housing like the ones described for northern Europe in the Introduction.

Records from New York City in the 1800s show repeated epidemics until about 1901 (Fig. 1–2). They included yellow fever, cholera, typhus fever, influenza and smallpox. Others not shown were scarlatina, thrush, diphtheria, whooping cough, measles, dysentery, pneumonia, bronchitis, tuberculosis, and syphilis.

Similarly, death records presented in Table 1–6 indicate the toll taken by tuberculosis, typhoid, diptheria, and smallpox during the 1800s in Massachusetts. Mortality information obtained in the 1850 census shows that as many as 50% of the deaths in several states and urban areas were due to such infectious diseases.

Death rates for major causes from 1900 to 1982 are shown in Table 1–7. The leading killers in 1900 were cardiovascular/renal disease, influenza/pneumonia, tuberculosis, gastritis, and other digestive-tract ailments. Most of the epidemics subsided in the late 1800s, but the complex of infectious diseases, including tuberculosis, pneumonia, influenza, and bronchitis was a leading cause of death until the 1920s. In 1918, influenza/pnuemonia was

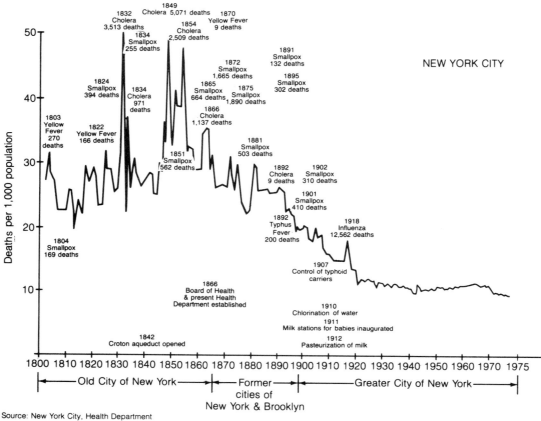

FIG. 1–2.   Mortality transition in New York City

Source: New York City, Health Department

the leading cause of death, with 588.2 deaths per 100,000 registered. By 1949, the rate of death due to this cause had fallen to only 30.0, a stabilization level where it has remained for most years since then. As of the late 1970s, the proportion of deaths from infectious disease was down from 50% to 6%, and cardiovascular disease had moved up to the number one killer in the United States (Table 1–7).

Changes in the cause of death in the United States since 1950 are graphically depicted in Fig. 1–3. It shows a mild continued decline in mortality from influenza/pneumonia since 1970 and a steady decline in heart disease and cerebrovascular diseases since 1950. The same is true of atherosclerosis. Deaths from diabetes have been falling since 1950 with one limited interruption.

Cancer mortality and obstructive pulmonary disease increased through 1983; homicides and suicides have been rising from 1950

TABLE 1–6. Death Rate, by Sex and by Selected Cause, for Massachusetts: 1860–1970 (Includes only deaths, excluding fetal deaths, occurring within Massachusetts, except for 1940–1970; for these years, data are for deaths occurring to residents of Massachusetts)

YEAR	By Sex per 1,000 Population			By Cause per 100,000 Population				
	Total	Male	Female	Tuberculosis of respiratory system	Diptheria	Typhoid and paratyphoid fever*	Measles	Smallpox
	193	194	195	196	197	198	199	200
1970	10.1	.....	.....	2.4	–†	(Z)	(Z)	....
1969	10.6	.....	.....	2.4	.	(Z)	(Z)	....
1968	10.9	.....	.....	2.9	.	(Z)	–	....
1967	10.7	.....	.....	3.5	.	(Z)	–	....
1966	10.7	.....	.....	3.3	.	(Z)	–	....
1965	11.0	.....	.....	4.0	.	(Z)	0.1	....
1964	9.6‡	.....	.....	3.3	.	(Z)	(Z)	....
1963	10.5	.....	.....	4.4	(Z)	(Z)	–	....
1962	10.8	.....	.....	4.8	.	(Z)	–	....
1961	10.8	.....	.....	5.7	.	0.1	(Z)	....
1960	11.0	.....	.....	6.0	.	(Z)	–	....
1959	10.7	.....	.....	6.6	.	(Z)	.	....
1958	11.3	.....	.....	6.5	.	(Z)	–	....
1957	11.1	.....	.....	8.2	(Z)	.	–	....
1956	10.9	.....	.....	8.6	0.1	.	(Z)	(Z)
1955	10.9	.....	.....	9.3	(Z)	(Z)	.4	(Z)
1950	10.5	11.6	9.5	20.2	.2	.1	.2	(Z)
1945	12.2	(NA)	(NA)	36.9	.3	.2	.2	(Z)
1940	11.9	12.6	11.1	34.6	.2	.3	.3	(Z)
1935	11.5	12.2	10.8	42.9	.7	.	.8	(Z)
1930	11.6	12.2	11.1	57.2	4.3	.9	3.3	(Z)
1925	12.5	13.0	11.9	70.1	8.0	1.8	8.4	(Z)
1920	13.8	13.9	13.6	96.8	15.1	2.4	9.1	.1
1915	14.3	15.0	13.7	116.8	19.8	6.7	7.3	.3
1910	16.1	17.0	15.3	138.3	21.0	12.5	11.6	(Z)
1905	16.7	17.6	15.8	163.5	22.1	17.9	8.4	.1
1900	18.4	19.2	17.6	190.3	52.8	22.1	11.7	.1
1899	17.4	(NA)	(NA)	190.4	38.2	22.3	8.8	.5
1898	17.5	(NA)	(NA)	197.4	26.4	24.7	3.1	(Z)
1897	18.1	(NA)	(NA)	207.4	54.5	23.2	6.0	.2
1896	19.3	(NA)	(NA)	216.4	65.5	28.3	5.4	(Z)
1895	19.0	19.9	18.2	223.4	71.4	27.2	4.7	(Z)
1894	19.1	(NA)	(NA)	223.4	73.6	30.6	4.0	1.3
1893	20.5	(NA)	(NA)	231.0	58.3	31.4	11.5	.4
1892	20.9	(NA)	(NA)	244.8	62.2	35.3	3.8	0.1
1891	19.7	(NA)	(NA)	239.6	53.2	35.9	10.3	.1
1890	19.4	20.0	18.9	258.6	72.6	37.3	5.1	(Z)
1889	19.2	(NA)	(NA)	256.5	101.7	40.9	7.9	.3
1888	19.9	(NA)	(NA)	270.8	86.6	44.6	10.4	.4
1887	19.8	(NA)	(NA)	285.6	79.2	44.8	22.1	.1
1886	18.6	(NA)	(NA)	295.1	78.0	40.0	6.5	(Z)
1885	19.6	20.2	19.0	306.6	78.4	39.5	16.1	1.0
1884	19.0	(NA)	(NA)	303.6	86.2	45.8	3.9	.2
1883	20.1	(NA)	(NA)	316.0	86.4	45.8	17.1	.3
1882	19.9	(NA)	(NA)	317.9	96.0	58.5	3.7	2.4
1881	20.1	(NA)	(NA)	324.5	131.4	59.1	12.7	2.6
1880	19.8	20.3	19.3	308.1	134.3	49.5	13.2	2.1
1879	18.1	(NA)	(NA)	297.4	130.6	36.3	1.1	.4
1878	18.1	(NA)	(NA)	308.4	145.5	39.3	17.6	.1
1877	18.4	(NA)	(NA)	320.4	186.6	47.8	7.9	1.4
1876	19.8	(NA)	(NA)	317.6	196.4	52.5	2.8	1.8
1875	21.7	21.8	20.5	347.4	113.8	64.1	14.1	2.1
1874	18.6	(NA)	(NA)	328.0	56.7	71.2	10.0	1.6
1873	21.6	(NA)	(NA)	353.6	47.4	89.5	11.5	42.5
1872	22.9	(NA)	(NA)	362.6	49.1	111.1	27.9	67.2
1871	18.7	(NA)	(NA)	339.3	50.0	74.7	8.8	19.7
1870	18.8	19.5	18.6	343.3	46.4	91.5	18.5	9.0
1869	18.4	(NA)	(NA)	328.8	54.3	85.0	15.7	4.2
1868	18.6	(NA)	(NA)	322.0	56.7	65.0	20.8	1.5
1867	17.0	(NA)	(NA)	325.5	45.3	72.0	14.5	14.6
1866	18.2	(NA)	(NA)	353.0	63.7	83.7	8.4	10.8
1865	20.6	21.7	19.6	367.9	92.8	133.7	10.7	17.4
1864	22.8	(NA)	(NA)	375.7	158.7	106.7	25.4	19.2
1863	22.2	(NA)	(NA)	372.6	182.4	115.1	11.3	3.4
1862	18.5	(NA)	(NA)	342.8	92.1	91.1	29.6	3.2
1861	19.5	(NA)	(NA)	365.2	89.2	79.9	16.9	2.7
1860	18.7	19.3	18.4	......	68.0	76.1	18.2	27.1

*Beginning 1958, includes "other salmonella infections."
†Represents zero
NA, Not available
Z, Less than 0.05
‡Excludes approximately 6,000 deaths registered in Massachusetts, primarily to residents of the State.
Source: *Colonial Statistics of the United States*

TABLE 1–7.   Death Rate, for Selected Causes: 1900–1970, 1982 (Number of deaths, excluding fetal deaths, per 100,000 population. Prior to 1933, for death-registration area only)

YEAR	Tuberculosis, All Forms	Syphilis and its Sequelae*	Typhoid and Paratyphoid Fever	Scarlet Fever and Streptococcal Sore Throat	Hepatitis	Diphtheria	Whooping Cough	Measles
	149	150	151	152	153	154	155	156
1982	0.8	(Z)	0.0	(Z)	0.3	(Z)	—	—
1970	2.6	0.2	(Z)	(Z)	0.5	(Z)	(Z)	(Z)
1969	2.8	.3	(Z)	(Z)	.5	(Z)	(Z)	(Z)
1968	3.1	.3	(Z)	(Z)	.4	(Z)	(Z)	(Z)
1967	3.5	1.2	(Z)	(Z)	.4	(Z)	(Z)	(Z)
1966	3.9	1.1	(Z)	(Z)	.4	(Z)	(Z)	.1
1965	4.1	1.3	(Z)	(Z)	.4	(Z)	(Z)	.1
1964	4.3	1.4	(Z)	(Z)	.4	(Z)	(Z)	.2
1963	4.9	1.4	(Z)	(Z)	.5	(Z)	(Z)	.2
1962	5.1	1.5	(Z)	(Z)	.5	(Z)	(Z)	.2
1961	5.4	1.6	(Z)	.1	.5	(Z)	(Z)	.2
1960§	6.1	1.6	(Z)	.1	.5	(Z)	.1	.2
1959$	6.5	1.7	(Z)	.1	.5	(Z)	.2	.2
1958	7.1	2.0	(Z)	.1	.5	(Z)	.1	.3
1957	7.8	2.2	(Z)	.1	.5	(Z)	.1	.2
1956	8.4	2.3	(Z)	.1	.5	.1	.2	.3
1955	9.1	2.3	(Z)	.1	.5	.1	.3	.2
1954	10.2	3.0	(Z)	.1	.5	.1	.2	.3
1953	12.3	3.3	(Z)	.1	.5	.1	.2	.3
1952	15.8	3.7	.1	.2	.5	.1	.3	.4
1951	20.1	4.1	.1	.2	.4	.2	.6	.4
1950	22.5	5.0	.1	.2	.4	.3	.7	.3
1949	26.3	5.8	.1	.3	.4	.4	.5	.6
1948	30.0	8.0	.2	(Z)	....	.4	.8	.6
1947	33.5	8.8	.2	.1	....	.6	1.4	.3
1946	36.4	9.3	.3	.1	....	.9	.9	.9
1945	39.9	10.6	.4	.2	....	1.2	1.3	.2
1944	41.2	11.2	.4	.3	....	.9	1.4	1.4
1943	42.5	12.1	.5	.3	....	.9	2.5	1.0
1942	43.1	12.2	.6	.3	....	1.0	1.9	1.0
1941	44.5	13.3	.8	.3	....	1.0	2.8	1.7
1940	45.9	14.4	1.1	.5	....	1.1	2.2	.5
1939	47.1	15.0	1.5	.7	....	1.5	2.3	.9
1938	49.1	15.9	1.9	.9	....	2.0	3.7	2.5
1937	53.8	16.1	2.1	1.4	....	2.0	3.9	1.2
1936	55.9	16.2	2.5	1.9	....	2.4	2.1	1.0
1935	55.1	15.4	2.8	2.1	....	3.1	3.7	3.1
1934	56.7	15.9	3.4	2.0	....	3.3	5.9	5.5
1933	59.6	15.1	3.6	2.0	....	3.9	3.6	2.2
1932	62.5	15.4	3.7	2.2	....	4.4	4.5	1.6
1931	67.8	15.4	4.5	2.2	....	4.8	3.9	3.0
1930	71.1	15.7	4.8	1.9	....	4.9	4.8	3.2
1929	75.3	15.6	4.2	2.1	....	6.5	6.2	2.5
1928	78.3	16.4	4.9	1.9	....	7.2	5.4	5.2
1927	79.6	16.4	5.3	2.3	....	7.7	6.8	4.1
1926	85.5	17.1	6.4	2.5	....	7.4	8.8	8.3
1925	84.8	17.3	7.8	2.7	....	7.8	6.7	2.3
1924	87.9	17.8	6.6	3.1	....	9.3	8.1	8.2
1923	91.7	17.9	6.7	3.5	....	12.0	9.6	10.7
1922	95.3	18.0	7.4	3.5	....	14.6	5.5	4.3
1921	97.6	17.5	8.8	5.3	....	17.7	9.1	4.2
1920	113.1	16.5	7.6	4.6	....	15.3	12.5	8.8
1919	125.6	16.2	9.2	2.8	....	14.9	5.6	3.9
1918	149.8	18.7	12.3	3.1	....	14.0	17.0	10.8

TABLE 1–7   (Continued)

Malignant Neoplasms[†]	Diabetes Mellitus	Major Cardiovascular-renal Diseases	Influenza and Pneumonia[‡]	Gastritis, Duodenitis Enteritis, and Colitis★★	Cirrhosis of Liver	Motor Vehicle Accidents[¶]	Accidental Falls	All Other Accidents[§]	Suicide
157	158	159	160	161	162	163	164	165	166
187.0	14.3	418.9	21.0	NA	11.7	19.6	NA	21.4	11.7
162.8	18.9	496.0	30.9	0.6	15.5	26.9	8.3	21.2	11.6
160.0	19.1	501.7	33.9	.9	14.8	27.6	8.8	21.2	11.1
159.4	19.2	512.1	36.8	.3	14.6	27.5	9.3	20.7	10.7
157.2	17.7	511.5	28.8	3.8	14.1	26.7	10.2	20.2	10.8
155.1	17.7	521.4	32.5	3.9	13.6	27.1	10.2	20.7	10.9
153.5	17.1	516.4	31.9	4.1	12.8	25.4	10.3	20.1	11.1
151.3	16.9	514.3	31.1	4.3	12.1	24.5	9.9	19.8	10.8
151.3	17.2	527.3	37.5	4.4	11.9	23.1	10.2	20.1	11.0
149.9	16.8	521.2	32.3	4.4	11.7	22.0	10.5	19.8	10.9
149.4	16.4	511.4	30.1	4.3	11.3	20.8	10.2	19.4	10.4
149.2	16.7	521.8	37.3	4.4	11.3	21.3	10.6	20.4	10.6
147.3	15.9	515.9	31.2	4.4	10.9	21.5	10.6	20.1	10.6
146.8	15.9	523.5	33.1	4.5	10.8	21.3	10.5	20.4	10.7
148.6	16.0	523.4	35.8	4.7	11.3	22.7	12.1	21.1	9.8
147.8	15.7	510.5	28.2	4.5	10.7	23.7	12.1	20.9	10.0
146.5	15.5	506.0	27.1	4.7	10.2	23.4	12.3	21.2	10.2
145.6	15.6	495.1	25.4	4.9	10.1	22.1	12.3	21.5	10.1
144.7	16.3	514.8	33.0	5.4	10.4	24.0	13.0	23.1	10.1
143.3	16.4	511.9	29.7	5.6	10.2	24.3	13.5	24.0	10.0
140.5	16.3	513.2	31.4	5.2	9.8	24.1	13.9	24.5	10.4
139.8	16.2	510.8	31.3	5.1	9.2	23.1	13.8	23.7	11.4
138.8	16.9	502.1	30.0	6.7	9.2	21.3	15.0	24.3	11.4
134.9	26.4	488.0	38.7	6.0	11.3	22.1	16.6	28.2	11.2
132.3	26.2	491.0	43.1	5.6	10.4	22.8	16.7	29.7	11.5
130.0	24.8	476.8	44.5	5.8	9.6	23.9	16.1	29.8	11.5
134.0	26.5	508.2	51.6	8.7	9.5	21.2	17.7	33.2	11.2
128.8	26.3	500.5	61.6	9.9	8.6	18.3	17.0	36.0	10.0
124.3	27.1	510.8	67.1	9.6	9.3	17.7	18.0	37.7	10.2
122.0	25.4	479.5	55.7	8.8	9.4	21.1	16.6	33.5	12.0
120.1	25.4	475.3	63.8	10.5	8.9	30.0	16.7	29.2	12.8
120.3	26.6	485.7	70.3	10.3	8.6	26.2	17.2	29.8	14.4
117.5	25.5	466.3	75.7	11.6	8.3	24.7	17.5	28.1	14.1
114.9	23.9	456.8	80.4	14.3	8.3	25.1	19.5	27.2	15.3
112.4	23.7	454.6	114.9	14.7	8.5	30.8	20.4	30.0	15.0
111.4	23.7	461.1	119.6	16.4	8.3	29.7	20.8	34.9	14.3
108.2	22.3	431.2	104.2	14.1	7.9	28.6	19.2	30.1	14.3
106.4	22.2	430.0	96.9	18.4	7.7	28.6	18.8	32.0	14.9
102.3	21.4	413.6	95.7	17.3	7.4	25.0	15.1	31.8	15.9
102.3	22.0	418.2	107.3	16.1	7.2	23.6	14.8	32.4	17.4
99.0	20.4	407.1	107.5	20.5	7.4	27.1	14.6	36.1	16.8
97.4	19.1	414.4	102.5	26.0	7.2	26.7	14.7	38.4	15.6
95.8	18.8	418.9	146.5	23.3	7.2	25.5	14.5	39.7	13.9
95.7	19.0	419.1	142.5	26.4	7.5	23.2	14.1	40.8	13.5
95.2	17.4	398.3	102.2	27.1	7.4	21.6	14.0	41.5	13.2
94.6	17.9	410.6	141.7	32.9	7.2	19.9	14.0	43.3	12.6
92.0	16.8	391.5	121.7	38.6	7.2	16.8	13.4	46.3	12.0
90.4	16.4	383.4	115.2	33.7	7.3	15.3	13.1	45.4	11.9
88.4	17.7	380.8	151.7	39.1	7.1	14.6	12.8	46.9	11.5
86.2	18.3	366.6	132.3	38.9	7.4	12.4	12.1	43.8	11.7
85.5	16.7	351.2	98.7	50.7	7.3	11.3	11.4	44.1	12.4
83.4	16.1	364.9	207.3	53.7	7.1	10.3	11.8	47.9	10.2
81.0	15.0	348.6	223.0	55.2	7.9	9.3	11.3	50.5	11.5
80.8	16.1	387.0	588.5	72.2	9.6	9.3	12.7	59.5	12.3

TABLE 1–7.   (Continued)

YEAR	Tuberculosis, All Forms	Syphilis and its Sequelae*	Typhoid and Paratyphoid Fever	Scarlet Fever and Streptococcal Sore Throat	Hepatitis	Diphtheria	Whooping Cough	Measles
	149	150	151	152	153	154	155	156
1917	143.5	19.1	13.3	3.5	....	15.6	10.5	14.1
1916	138.4	18.6	13.2	3.1	....	13.9	10.5	11.4
1915	140.1	17.7	11.8	3.6	....	15.2	8.2	5.2
1914	141.7	16.7	14.7	6.6	....	17.2	10.2	6.8
1913	143.5	16.2	17.5	7.7	....	18.1	10.1	12.8
1912	145.4	15.1	16.1	6.0	....	17.6	9.2	7.2
1911	155.1	15.3	20.1	8.6	....	18.4	11.0	9.9
1910	153.8	13.5	22.5	11.4	....	21.1	11.6	12.4
1909	156.3	12.9	20.2	11.1	....	19.9	10.0	10.0
1908	162.1	12.4	23.4	12.4	....	21.9	10.7	10.6
1907	174.2	12.4	28.2	9.3	....	24.2	11.3	9.6
1906	175.8	14.1	30.9	7.3	....	26.3	16.1	12.9
1905	179.9	13.8	22.4	6.8	....	23.5	8.9	7.4
1904	188.1	13.9	23.9	11.6	....	29.3	5.8	11.3
1903	177.2	13.2	24.6	12.3	....	31.1	14.3	8.8
1902	174.2	12.9	26.4	11.9	....	29.8	12.4	9.3
1901	189.9	12.5	27.6	13.6	....	33.5	8.7	7.4
1900	194.4	12.0	31.3	9.6	....	40.3	12.2	13.3

★1900–1920, excludes aneurysm of the aorta.
†Includes neoplasms of lymphatic and hematopoietic tissues.
‡All years, excludes pneumonia of newborn; 1900–1920, excludes capillary bronchitis.
★★All years, excludes diarrhea of newborn; 1900–1920, includes ulcer of duodenum.
¶¶1906–1925, excludes automobile collisions with trains and streetcars, and motorcycle accidents.
‖1900–1921, includes legal executions; 1900–1908, food poisoning; and 1900–1905 motor vehicle accidents.
§Denotes first year for which figures include Alaska and Hawaii.
$Includes Alaska.
Source: *Colonial Statistics of the United States*

through the 1980s. Oddly, the sharpest and steadiest mortality increase is from septicemia, the 14th leading cause of death in 1983. About 5% of hospitalized patients, or 175,000 patients acquire a noscomial infection annually and the estimated direct cost is more than $1 billion. This is particularly startling since septicemia is treatable by antibiotics available since 1950.

Some suggested explanations for the rise in septicemia deaths include increasing bacterial resistance to some of the common broad-spectrum antibiotics such as penicillin. Also, immunosuppressive drugs used to treat patients with certain conditions leave them susceptible to infection. Attention directed to individual outbreaks of infection among one or several hospital patients at the same institution has also revealed that such outbreaks occur because of lack of proper sanitary precautions taken by institutions, including the understerilization of surgical instruments and poor general housekeeping.

TABLE 1–7 (Continued)

Malignant Neoplasms[†]	Diabetes Mellitus	Major Cardiovascular-renal Diseases	Influenza and Pneumonia[‡]	Gastritis, Duodenitis Enteritis, and Colitis**	Cirrhosis of Liver	Motor Vehicle Accidents[†]	Accidental Falls	All Other Accidents[ǀ]	Suicide
157	158	159	160	161	162	163	164	165	166
80.8	16.9	396.4	164.5	75.2	10.9	8.6	14.8	62.6	13.0
81.0	16.9	389.4	163.3	75.5	11.8	7.1	15.1	59.4	13.7
80.7	17.6	383.5	145.9	67.5	12.1	5.8	14.8	52.9	16.2
78.7	16.2	374.5	132.4	75.1	12.5	4.2	15.0	57.5	16.1
78.5	15.4	370.6	140.8	86.7	12.9	3.8	15.4	64.5	15.4
77.0	15.1	375.7	138.4	79.6	13.1	2.8	15.4	62.6	15.6
74.2	15.1	366.5	145.4	86.8	13.6	2.1	15.0	66.5	16.0
76.2	15.3	371.9	155.9	115.4	13.3	1.8	15.4	67.0	15.3
74.0	14.1	362.0	148.1	101.8	13.4	1.2	....	77.5	16.0
71.5	13.8	356.7	150.9	112.5	13.5	.8	....	82.1	16.8
71.4	14.2	389.8	180.0	115.0	14.8	.7	....	94.1	14.5
69.3	13.4	364.3	156.3	123.6	14.1	.4	....	94.0	12.8
73.4	14.1	384.0	169.3	118.4	14.0	....		81.3	13.5
71.5	14.2	388.8	192.1	111.5	13.9	....		85.4	12.2
70.0	12.7	364.4	169.3	100.3	13.5	....		81.4	11.3
66.3	11.7	349.8	161.3	104.9	13.0	....		72.5	10.3
66.4	11.6	347.7	197.2	118.5	13.1	....		83.8	10.4
64.0	11.0	345.2	202.2	142.7	12.5	....		72.3	10.2

Today, almost as many people die in motor-vehicle accidents as from influenza/pneumonia, whereas malignant neoplasms (cancer) have become the second leading cause of death. The death rates for the major causes of death in the United States are compared to the rates for these same diseases in other countries (Table 1–9). Extreme variations from country to country are readily seen when the death-rate data for ischemic heart disease in which heart bloodflow is obstructed is compared for Japan and the United States. Dietary differences are suspected as a major cause for this difference. Table 1–10 shows that white American females in 1950 had a lower death rate than white males for each of the major causes of death except breast disease and diabetes. But by 1980, white females had a lower mortality rate for diabetes than white males. This left only breast cancer as a cause of greater mortality in white females than in males.

In 1950, black females had a higher mortality than black males from several diseases, including cerebrovascular disease, neoplasms, and diabetes. But by 1960, black females had a lower cerebrovascular death rate than black males. Between 1960 and 1980, the death rate from neoplasms fell among black females, whereas it rose among black males who reached a higher rate than black

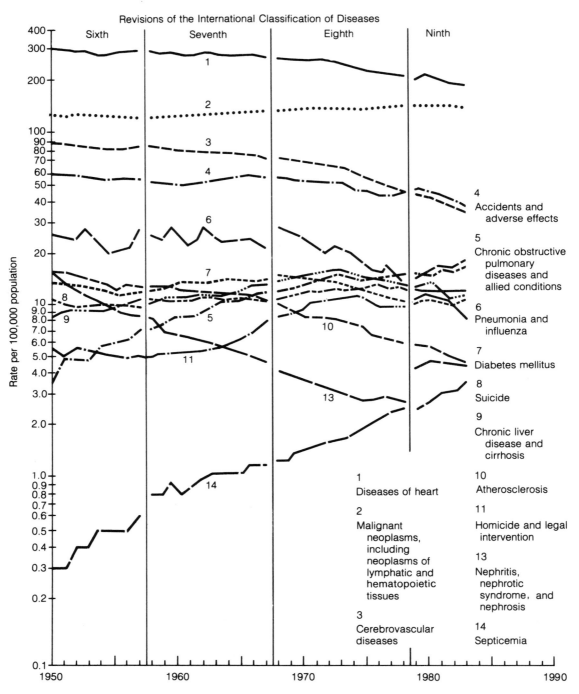

Revisions of the International Classification of Diseases

Source: *Monthly Vital Statistics Report,* Vol. 33, No. 9 Dec. 1984

TABLE 1–8.   Rates for 15 Leading Causes of Death: United States, 1981, 1982 (Based on a 10% sample of deaths, rates per 100,000 population)

RANK	Cause of Death (Ninth Revision International Classification of Diseases, 1975)	1981 Death rate	1982	1981 % of total deaths	1982
...	All causes	866.4	854.6	100.0	
1	Diseases of heart	330.6	325.7	38.2	38.1
2	Malignant neoplasms, including neoplasms of lymphatic and hematopoietic tissues	184.3	188.2	21.3	22.0
3	Cerebrovascular diseases	71.7	68.6	8.3	8.2
4	Accidents and adverse effects	44.5	40.9	5.1	4.8
...	Motor vehicle accidents	22.8	19.8	2.6	2.3
...	All other accidents and adverse effects	21.7	21.4	2.5	2.5
5	Chronic obstructive pulmonary diseases and allied conditions	26.1	25.5	3.0	3.0
6	Pheumonia and influenza	23.7	21.0	2.7	2.5
7	Diabetes mellitus	15.2	14.2	1.7	1.7
8	Chronic liver disease and cirrhosis	12.9	11.7	1.5	1.4
9	Atherosclerosis	12.5	11.4	1.4	1.3
10	Suicide	12.3	11.6	1.4	1.4
11	Homicide and legal intervention	10.7	9.5	1.2	1.1
12	Certain perinatal conditions	9.2	9.1	1.1	1.1
13	Nephritis, nephrotic syndrome, and nephrosis	7.6	8.0	0.9	0.9
14	Congenital anomalies	5.8	5.6	0.7	0.6
15	Septicemia	4.4	4.9	0.5	0.5
...	All other causes	94.9	—	10.9	—

Source: *Monthly Vital Statistics Report,* Vol. 30, No. 13, Dec. 1982

TABLE 1–9.   Deaths from Selected Causes for Selected Countries–Age-adjusted Rates: 1970–1979 [Deaths per 100,000 population; table is based on the sum of male and female population of 46 countries for which the source published causes of death statistics in 1950. Causes of death are classified according to eighth revision of the *International Classification of Diseases*]

SEX AND CAUSE OF DEATH	United States	Canada	France	Germany, Federal Republic	Japan	Sweden	United Kingdom⋆
Male:							
Ischemic heart disease:							
1970	319.7	272.9	68.7	153.5	49.2	224.9	241.3
1975	281.8	253.2	77.6	172.3	44.5	238.5	248.6
1979	261.6[†]	243.3[‡]	72.8[‡]	175.1[†]	39.0	244.9	243.5
Malignant neoplasms:							
1970	154.9	155.1	175.9	175.4	148.7	129.8	187.4
1975	159.1	158.0	189.0	181.8	140.3	146.3	184.9
1979	163.7[†]	159.1[‡]	193.3[‡]	181.3[†]	145.6	143.8	185.4
Cerebrovascular diseases:							
1970	75.8	65.9	93.1	109.0	214.8	55.7	92.5
1975	64.0	61.3	84.2	95.4	167.0	57.5	81.7
1979	53.1[†]	54.8[‡]	71.4[‡]	86.6[†]	128.4	49.8	73.8

TABLE 1–9. (Continued)

SEX AND CAUSE OF DEATH	United States	Canada	France	Germany, Federal Republic	Japan	Sweden	United Kingdom★
Male:							
Accidents:							
1970	78.0	75.0	82.4	76.5	65.5	46.5	37.6
1975	65.7	74.6	72.0	61.2	45.3	58.8	32.5
1979	64.5[†]	64.2[‡]	71.5[‡]	54.6[†]	36.7	52.1	31.3
Female:							
Ischemic heart disease:							
1970	163.9	132.9	28.8	63.3	28.1	120.4	101.3
1975	140.6	118.1	31.8	74.8	26.9	120.1	105.7
1979	132.8[†]	112.5[‡]	29.4[‡]	75.4[†]	22.6	112.2	100.9
Malignant neoplasms:							
1970	106.5	109.9	96.0	123.4	91.7	106.9	118.0
1975	105.2	105.8	96.2	119.4	87.0	110.7	119.9
1979	107.5[†]	105.7[‡]	93.5[‡]	116.6[†]	85.2	107.1	122.0
Cerebrovascular diseases:							
1970	65.4	57.1	65.0	87.2	142.5	51.1	82.4
1975	54.6	51.7	61.0	75.9	115.5	51.9	73.7
1979	46.7[†]	45.8[‡]	52.6[‡]	68.7[†]	90.5	42.8	67.3
Accidents:							
1970	28.8	29.0	35.1	31.9	26.8	20.1	18.5
1975	23.7	29.0	32.1	27.2	14.7	20.0	15.9
1979	23.8[†]	24.9[‡]	32.2[‡]	24.5[†]	12.9	17.7	15.1

★Covers England and Wales only
[†]1978 data
[‡]1977 data
Source: World Health Organization, Geneva, Switzerland, *World Health Statistics*, vol 1, annual.

TABLE 1–10. Age-adjusted Death Rates for Selected Causes of Death, According to Sex and Race: United States, Selected Years 1950–84 (Data are based on the National Vital Statistics System)

SEX, RACE, AND CAUSE OF DEATH	1950*	1960*	1970	1980	1981	1982	1983	1984*,[†]
All races:			Deaths per 100,000 resident population					
All causes	841.5	760.9	714.3	585.8	568.2	553.8	550.5	547.7
Diseases of heart	307.6	286.2	253.6	202.0	195.0	190.5	188.8	183.3
Cerebrovascular diseases	88.8	79.7	66.3	40.8	38.1	35.8	34.4	33.9
Malignant neoplasms	125.4	125.8	129.9	132.8	131.6	132.5	132.6	133.1
Respiratory system	12.8	19.2	28.4	36.4	36.6	37.5	37.9	38.5
Colorectal	19.0	17.7	16.8	15.5	15.1	15.0	14.9	—
Stomach	14.1	9.3	5.9	4.3	4.2	4.1	4.0	—
Breast[‡]	22.2	22.3	23.1	22.7	22.7	22.8	22.7	23.4
Chronic obstructive pulmonary diseases	4.4	8.2	13.2	15.9	16.3	16.2	17.4	18.0
Pneumonia and influenza	26.2	28.0	22.1	12.9	12.3	10.9	11.8	12.2
Chronic liver disease and cirrhosis	8.5	10.5	14.7	12.2	11.4	10.5	10.2	9.8
Diabetes mellitus	14.3	13.6	14.1	10.1	9.8	9.6	9.9	9.9
Accidents and adverse effects	57.5	49.9	53.7	42.3	39.8	36.6	35.3	35.6
Motor vehicle accidents	23.3	22.5	27.4	22.9	21.8	19.3	18.5	19.2

TABLE 1–10.   (Continued)

SEX, RACE, AND CAUSE OF DEATH	1950*	1960*	1970	1980	1981	1982	1983	1984*,†
All races:	Deaths per 100,000 resident population							
Suicide	11.0	10.6	11.8	11.4	11.5	11.6	11.4	11.6
Homicide and legal intervention	5.4	5.2	9.1	10.8	10.4	9.7	8.6	8.2
White Male:								
All causes	963.1	917.7	893.4	745.3	724.4	706.0	698.4	694.6
Diseases of heart	381.1	375.4	347.6	277.5	268.8	262.1	257.8	—
Cerebrovascular diseases	87.0	80.3	68.8	41.9	38.9	36.6	35.2	—
Malignant neoplasms	130.9	141.6	154.3	160.5	158.3	159.4	158.9	—
Respiratory system	21.6	34.6	49.9	58.0	57.8	58.5	58.0	—
Colorectal	19.8	18.9	18.9	18.3	17.9	17.7	17.8	—
Stomach	17.8	11.9	7.7	5.6	5.6	5.3	5.1	—
Chronic obstructive pulmonary diseases	6.0	13.8	24.0	26.7	26.8	26.2	27.6	—
Pneumonia and influenza	27.1	31.0	26.0	16.2	15.6	14.3	15.3	—
Chronic liver disease and cirrhosis	11.6	14.4	18.8	15.7	14.8	14.1	13.4	—
Diabetes mellitus	11.3	11.6	12.7	9.5	9.3	9.2	9.2	—
Accidents and adverse effects	80.9	70.5	76.2	62.3	59.1	54.1	51.8	—
Motor vehicle accidents	35.9	34.0	40.1	34.8	33.4	29.3	27.8	—
Suicide	18.1	17.5	18.2	18.9	18.9	19.4	19.3	—
Homicide and legal intervention	3.9	3.9	7.3	10.9	10.3	9.5	8.4	—
Black male:								
All causes	1,373.1	1,246.1	1,318.6	1,112.8	1,067.7	1,035.0	1,019.6	1,016.1
Diseases of heart	415.5	381.2	375.9	327.3	316.7	309.4	308.2	—
Cerebrovascular diseases	146.2	141.2	124.2	77.5	72.7	68.9	64.2	—
Malignant neoplasms	126.1	158.5	198.0	229.9	232.0	235.2	232.2	—
Respiratory system	16.9	36.6	60.8	82.0	84.1	85.8	83.3	—
Colorectal	13.8	15.0	17.3	19.2	19.1	19.6	19.0	—
Stomach	25.7	20.8	15.5	11.1	11.1	11.5	11.0	—
Chronic obstructive pulmonary diseases	—	—	—	20.9	21.4	20.6	22.2	—
Pneumonia and influenza	63.8	70.2	53.8	28.0	26.4	23.2	24.3	—
Chronic liver disease and cirrhosis	8.8	14.8	33.1	30.6	27.3	23.5	22.8	—
Diabetes mellitus	11.5	16.2	21.2	17.7	16.8	16.1	17.7	—
Accidents and adverse effects	105.7	100.0	119.5	82.0	74.7	68.3	66.2	—
Motor vehicle accidents	39.8	38.2	50.1	32.9	30.7	27.2	26.4	—
Suicide	7.0	7.8	9.9	11.1	11.0	10.8	10.5	—
Homicide and legal intervention	51.1	44.9	82.1	71.9	69.2	62.3	53.8	—
White Female:								
All causes	645.0	555.0	501.7	411.1	401.4	393.3	392.7	391.4
Diseases of heart	223.6	197.1	167.8	134.6	129.8	127.4	126.7	—
Cerebrovascular diseases	79.7	68.7	56.2	35.2	33.1	31.0	29.6	—
Malignant neoplasms	119.4	109.5	107.6	107.7	107.2	108.2	108.5	—
Respiratory system	4.6	5.1	10.1	18.2	18.8	20.0	21.0	—
Colorectal	19.0	17.0	15.3	13.3	12.9	12.7	12.5	—
Stomach	—	6.1	3.7	2.6	2.5	2.5	2.4	—
Breast	9.6	22.4	23.4	22.8	22.8	22.8	22.7	—
Chronic obstructive pulmonary disease	22.5	3.3	5.3	9.2	9.8	10.0	11.3	—
Pneumonia and influenza	2.8	19.0	15.0	9.4	9.0	7.6	8.6	—
Chronic liver disease and cirrhosis	18.9	6.6	8.7	7.0	6.7	6.1	6.0	—
Diabetes mellitus	5.8	13.7	12.8	8.7	8.4	8.3	8.6	—
Accidents and adverse effects	16.4	25.5	27.2	21.4	20.2	18.7	18.3	—
Motor vehicle accidents	30.6	11.1	14.4	12.3	11.7	10.5	10.3	—
Suicide	10.6	5.3	7.2	5.7	6.0	5.8	5.6	—
Homicide and legal intervention	5.3	1.5	2.2	3.2	3.1	3.1	2.8	—

TABLE 1–10.   (Continued)

SEX, RACE, AND CAUSE OF DEATH	1950*	1960*	1970	1980	1981	1982	1983	1984*,†
Black Female:	1.4							
All causes	1,106.7	916.9	814.4	631.1	599.1	581.4	590.4	586.2
Diseases of heart	349.5	292.6	251.7	201.1	191.2	186.3	191.5	—
Cerebrovascular diseases	155.6	139.5	107.9	61.7	58.1	54.7	53.8	—
Malignant neoplasms	131.9	127.8	123.5	129.7	127.1	128.7	129.8	—
Respiratory system	4.1	5.5	10.9	19.5	20.1	20.4	22.0	—
Colorectal	15.0	15.4	16.1	15.3	15.3	15.5	15.1	—
Stomach	13.1	9.1	6.0	4.8	5.0	4.4	4.7	—
Breast	19.3	21.3	21.5	23.3	23.7	24.6	24.4	—
Chronic obstructive pulmonary diseases	—	—	—	6.3	6.3	7.3	7.6	—
Pneumonia and influenza	50.4	43.9	29.2	12.7	11.3	10.1	10.2	—
Chronic liver disease and cirrhosis	5.7	8.9	17.8	14.4	12.7	10.9	10.8	—
Diabetes mellitus	22.7	27.3	30.9	22.1	21.3	19.8	21.1	—
Accidents and adverse effects	38.5	35.9	35.3	25.1	21.6	20.8	21.9	—
Motor vehicle accidents	10.3	10.0	13.8	8.4	7.7	7.5	7.5	—
Suicide	1.7	1.9	2.9	2.4	2.5	2.2	2.1	—
Homicide and legal intervention	11.7	11.8	15.0	13.7	12.9	12.0	11.2	—

*Includes deaths of nonresidents of the United States.
†Provisional data.
‡Female only.
Sources: National Center for Health Statistics: *Vital Statistics Rates in the United States, 1940–1960*, by R. D. Grove and A. M. Hetzel. DHEW Pub. No. (PHS) 1677. Public Health Service. Washington. U.S. Government Printing Office, 1968; Unpublished data from the Division of Vital Statistics; *Vital Statistics of the United States*, Vol II, Mortality, Part A, 1950–83. Public Health Service. Washington. U.S. Government Printing Office; Annual summary of births, deaths, marriages, and divorces, United States, 1984. *Monthly Vital Statistics Report*. Vol. 33-No. 13. DHHS Pub. No. (PHS) 84-1120. Public Health Service. Hyattsville, Md., Sept. 26, 1985; Data computed by the Division of Analysis from data compiled by the Division of Vital Statistics.

females. Only diabetes and breast disease remained as causes of greater mortality in black females compared to black males.

Most of the decline in mortality, however, reflects a fall in causes of death that struck particularly at the weak and susceptible, such as infants and children. The greatest gains in longevity have been for infants, children, and those who ministered to them when they suffered from communicable disease—young adult women. These same two populations gained from advances in child delivery, such as the widespread use of forceps and improved safety of cesarean section. More than others, their gain in longevity has boosted the average lifespan of the entire population. The same is true of other developed countries.

Analysis of the marked increase in average life expectancy at birth in developed countries such as the United States, is most directly accomplished by reviewing the drastic change in infant mortality rates that have occurred in the 20th century.

Infant Mortality And Morbidity 2

The infant mortality rate is calculated as the annual number of infant deaths per 1,000 live births during the same year. This rate is a rather crude measure: an infant dying in the first year of life may not die in the calendar year in which it is born. Still, this rate is a reasonable indicator if the level of live births is fairly constant from one calendar year to the next.

OVERALL RATE

By the late 1970s, the U.S. infant mortality rate had reached record lows. The 1981 rate, however, was still below that of 1980 at 11.5 per 1,000, down from 12.5 per 1,000. The 1983 rate of 10.6 per 1,000 was the lowest rate ever recorded, representing about 40,000 infant deaths nationally.

The U.S. infant mortality rate compared to that of other developed countries is summarized in Table 2–1. Although American medical technology is as advanced as it is elsewhere, the socio-economic mix in the U.S. population is greater than in several countries with lower infant mortality rates.

The difference in survival between white and non-white infants nationally is still substantial. Table 2–2 shows the mortality rate for infants born in the United States from 1915 to 1983 according

25

TABLE 2–1. Infant Mortality Rates and Average Annual Percentage Change: Selected Countries, 1977 and 1982 (Data are based on National Vital Statistics Systems)

	INFANT MORTALITY RATE*		Average Annual Change‡ (%)
COUNTRY	1977	1982†	
Finland	9.1	6.5	−8.1
Japan	8.9	6.6	−5.8
Sweden	8.0	6.8	−3.2
Norway	9.2	7.5	−5.0
Switzerland	9.8	7.6	−6.2
Netherlands	9.5	8.1	−3.1
Denmark	8.7	8.4	−0.7
Canada	12.4	9.6	−6.2
France	11.4	9.6	−4.2
Australia	12.5	10.0	−5.4
Spain	15.6	10.3	−9.9
Singapore	12.4	10.8	−2.7
United Kingdom	14.1	11.1	−5.8
United States	14.1	11.5	−4.0
Federal Republic of Germany	15.5	11.6	−7.0
Belgium	13.6	11.7	−3.7
New Zealand	14.2	11.8	−3.6
German Democratic Republic	13.1	12.3	−1.6
Austria	16.8	12.8	−5.3
Italy	18.1	14.1	−6.1
Greece	20.4	14.2	−8.7
Israel	18.2	15.6	−3.8
Czechoslovakia	19.7	16.1	−4.0
Jamaica	15.2	16.2	6.6
Cuba	23.5	17.3	−5.9

*Per 1,000 live births.
†Data for Jamaica are the 1978. Data for Finland, Norway, Switzerland, Canada, France, Australia, Spain, United Kingdom, Federal Republic of Germany, Belgium, German Democratic Republic, Italy, Greece, and Israel are for 1981. Data for all other countries refer to 1982; of these, the U.S. figure is final and all others are provisional.
‡Average annual percentage change is between 1977 and the most recent year data are available.
Note: Rankings are from lowest to highest infant mortality rates based on the latest data available for countries or geographic areas with at least 1 million population and with "complete" counts of live births and infant deaths as indicated in the United Nations Demographic Yearbook, 1982.
Sources: United Nations: Demographic Yearbook, 1981 and 1982. Pub. Nos.ST/ESA/STAT/SER.R/11 and ST/ESA/STAT/SER.R/12. New York. United Nations, 1983 and 1984; National Center for Health Statistics: Advance report of final mortality statistics, 1982, Monthly Vital Statistics Report. Vol. 33-No. 9, Supp. DHHS Pub. No. (PHS) 84-1120. Public Health Service. Hyattsville, Md., June 21. 1984.

TABLE 2–2. U.S. Infant Mortality by Race, 1915–1983

YEAR	Total	White	All other	Year	Total	White	All other
1983	10.8	9.4	26.8				
1982	11.5	10.1	17.3				
1981	11.7	10.6	17.3				
1980	12.5	10.8	20.7				
1979	13.1	11.4	22.6				
1978*	13.8	12.0	21.1	1956	26.0	23.2	42.1
1977*	14.1	12.3	21.7	1955	26.4	23.6	42.8
1975*	15.2	13.3	23.5	1954	26.6	23.9	42.9
1975*	16.1	14.2	24.2	1953	27.8	25.0	44.7
1974*	16.7	14.8	24.9	1952	28.4	25.5	47.0
1973*	17.7	15.8	26.2	1951	28.4	25.8	44.8

YEAR	Total	White	All other	Year	Total	White	All other
1972*†	18.5	16.4	27.7	1950	29.2	26.8	44.5
1971*	19.1	17.1	28.5	1949	31.3	28.9	47.3
1970*	20.0	17.8	30.9	1948	32.0	29.9	46.5
1969	20.9	18.4	32.9	1947	32.2	30.1	48.5
1968	21.8	19.2	34.5	1946	33.8	31.8	49.5
1967	22.4	19.7	35.9	1945	38.3	35.6	57.0
1966	23.7	20.6	38.8	1944	39.8	36.9	60.3
1965	24.7	21.5	40.3	1943	40.4	37.5	62.5
1964	24.8	21.6	41.1	1942	40.4	37.3	64.6
1963‡	25.2	22.2	41.5	1941	45.3	41.2	74.8
1962‡	25.3	22.3	41.4	1940	47.0	43.2	73.8
1961	25.3	22.4	40.7	1935-39	53.2	49.2	81.3
1960	26.0	22.9	43.2	1930-34**	60.4	55.2	98.6
1959	26.4	23.2	44.0	1925-29	69.0	65.0	105.4
1958	27.1	23.8	45.7	1920-24	76.7	73.3	115.3
1957	26.3	23.3	43.7	1915-19	95.7	92.8	149.7

*Excludes deaths of nonresidents of the United States.
†Deaths based on a 50-percent sample.
‡Figures by race exclude data for residents of New Jersey.
**For 1932-34. Mexicans are included with "All other."
Source: *Vital Statistics of the U.S., Mortality* 1981 Vol. II.

to their race (specified as "white" and "all other"). Indian infants have a slightly higher mortality rate than whites, whereas Oriental babies have a much lower one (Table 2–3). Thus, the grouping of Oriental and Indian infants in the "all other" category doesn't change the fact that the dramatic difference in mortality rates is really between black and white infants (see Table 1–2).

In 1956, the "all other" infant mortality rate was 80% higher than for whites. Despite advances since 1956, the "all other" rate—tantamount to a black rate—in 1983 was still almost 80% higher than the white rate at 16.8 vs. 9.4 per 1,000 live births.

The U.S. mortality rate for various minority infants for selected years is shown in Table 2–3. Since 1950, the Chinese and Japanese-American infant mortality rate has been substantially lower than it has been for white infants. Oddly, this striking fact has elicited little notice or comment.

The American Indian rate, the highest by far of any group in 1950, is now near that of white infants. Like white babies, however, Indian babies still have a much higher death rate than Oriental babies. The gains among the American Indian population are impressive; they've fallen from a rate twice as high as the one for blacks in 1950 to one that was only 65% of the black infant mortality rate by 1977.

The infant mortality rate within specific narrow age groupings younger than age 1 year for white and "all other" U.S. infants as

TABLE 2–3.   U.S. Infant Mortality by Minorities, 1950–1977

YEAR*	Black	American Indian	Chinese-American	Japanese-American	White
1950	43.9	82.1	19.3	19.1	26.8
1960	44.3	49.3	14.7	15.3	22.9
1970[†]	32.6	22.0	8.4	10.6	17.8
1977[†]	23.6	15.6	5.9	6.6	12.3

*Deaths of infants under 1 year of age per 1,000 live births.
[†]Excludes deaths of nonresidents of the United States.
Source: Public Health Reports Supplement to Sept./Oct. 1980

of 1982 is shown in Table 2–4. Again, while "all other" includes Oriental and American Indian infants, since 1970 their rates are near or better than those of whites (Table 2–3). Most of the differences between white infants and all others is, therefore, between whites and blacks (Table 2–4).

In view of this fact, it's important to note that the white–nonwhite difference is not as great for the neonatal period of 0 to 28 days as it is for the postneonatal period of 28 days through the seventh month. This supports the common contention that en-

TABLE 2–4.   Infant Mortality Rates by Age and Color: United States, 1969–78 and 1982*
[Rates per 100,000 live births in specified group]

COLOR AND AGE	1982	1978*	1977*	1976*	1975*	1974*	1973*	1972*,[†]	1971*	1970*	1969
Total											
Under 1 year	1,150	1,378.4	1,412.1	1,523.6	1,606.9	1,670.1	1,771.8	1,847.0	1,911.7	2,001.1	2,085.2
Under 28 days	770	948.6	987.8	1,091.8	1,158.2	1,225.9	1,296.3	1,363.6	1,420.0	1,508.3	1,557.8
Under 1 day		510.9	529.8	533.4	630.0	669.5	721.8	786.8	819.7	882.0	918.1
1 day		99.5	110.8	123.2	142.2	163.9	173.7	181.9	200.1	212.9	221.8
2 days		78.6	83.1	90.7	98.5	103.3	113.2	111.6	126.5	127.6	131.9
3 days		44.2	44.0	49.3	50.1	52.2	55.0	57.5	59.3	58.0	58.6
4 days		28.0	28.7	29.1	32.6	34.0	33.0	35.9	34.8	36.1	34.7
5 days		20.5	22.4	24.6	27.1	25.8	26.4	22.4	24.7	26.4	24.2
6 days		16.4	18.1	20.8	18.1	18.9	20.0	18.5	16.6	19.1	19.0
7–13 days		77.9	79.0	87.2	85.1	84.2	77.3	75.7	70.9	72.9	74.9
14–20 days		42.3	41.5	43.1	43.7	42.4	41.8	39.8	36.4	39.2	40.1
21–27 days		30.2	30.5	30.4	30.8	31.7	34.1	33.6	31.1	34.2	34.5
28–59 days		105.4	104.7	108.0	117.3	115.1	120.8	119.4	122.9	124.9	129.9
2 months		85.6	84.9	86.5	86.5	85.6	92.7	90.4	93.1	95.4	98.9
3 months		64.6	63.8	66.2	66.2	66.5	68.3	69.9	71.0	69.3	76.4
4 months		46.3	43.9	43.1	47.1	45.6	47.0	49.4	49.7	50.0	54.9
5 months		33.2	33.0	31.3	31.6	31.6	34.4	35.2	36.1	37.0	40.6
6 months		24.5	25.3	24.0	25.5	25.2	27.6	30.3	29.2	28.5	31.5
7 months		18.4	19.2	18.8	19.5	20.3	21.4	23.9	23.9	23.4	24.7
8 months		16.3	15.4	16.0	15.6	14.9	17.2	20.7	19.2	18.2	21.8
9 months		12.6	12.4	13.8	14.9	14.3	15.5	16.5	16.9	18.0	17.8
10 months		11.8	10.8	12.5	12.9	13.1	15.2	14.3	15.1	15.1	16.1
11 months		11.1	10.8	11.6	11.4	12.1	15.4	13.3	14.6	14.9	15.0

COLOR AND AGE	1982	1978*	1977*	1976*	1975*	1974*	1973*	1972*,†	1971*	1970*	1969
White:											
Under 1 year	1,010	1,201.4	1,233.7	1,330.5	1,417.4	1,484.9	1,577.4	1,636.6	1,707.1	1,775.2	1,840.9
Under 28 days	680	838.5	874.7	965.3	1,037.5	1,113.9	1,183.9	1,236.8	1,302.3	1,376.9	1,416.6
Under 1 day		440.0	464.3	516.8	558.0	603.0	652.7	709.9	747.6	798.5	827.7
1 day		89.0	99.2	110.4	128.2	150.0	161.5	169.2	187.3	197.7	208.8
2 days		71.3	77.1	83.7	91.4	99.6	109.3	105.1	121.9	123.4	128.2
3 days		41.6	41.4	46.1	47.4	48.8	50.6	52.9	56.0	54.7	56.3
4 days		26.4	26.1	26.6	29.9	32.3	31.0	33.2	31.2	32.8	31.1
5 days		18.6	19.6	21.0	24.7	22.9	24.2	20.7	21.6	24.1	21.5
6 days		15.0	16.9	19.0	16.8	16.7	17.5	16.5	14.9	17.2	16.9
7–13 days		73.3	69.8	79.0	77.3	77.1	71.3	68.0	64.3	66.3	64.9
14–20 days		37.8	35.4	37.3	37.9	37.5	36.8	33.6	31.5	34.0	33.9
21–27 days		25.5	25.3	25.9	25.7	26.1	29.1	27.6	26.0	28.3	28.4
28–59 days		87.8	86.5	89.1	98.0	94.5	98.5	97.8	101.5	101.9	104.2
2 months		70.9	70.9	72.6	74.1	70.0	75.9	76.7	76.0	76.5	79.2
3 months		54.2	54.4	56.7	54.6	57.8	56.6	58.6	59.7	56.1	61.6
4 months		39.4	37.5	36.5	39.3	36.5	38.5	38.6	40.8	40.2	43.5
5 months		27.7	28.1	26.3	26.7	25.7	28.5	27.9	28.4	28.6	31.6
6 months		20.4	21.0	19.8	22.1	21.8	23.1	25.7	23.5	22.9	24.9
7 months		16.1	17.2	16.8	16.2	18.3	17.8	20.5	20.0	18.4	20.4
8 months		14.2	13.2	13.8	13.9	12.8	14.4	16.8	15.8	15.2	17.9
9 months		11.3	10.8	11.5	13.1	12.2	13.8	14.5	13.5	13.3	14.8
10 months		10.5	9.7	11.1	12.0	11.5	12.9	11.7	13.2	12.7	13.9
11 months		10.4	9.5	10.6	9.9	10.0	13.6	11.0	12.4	12.5	12.2
All Other:											
Under 1 year	1,730	2,105.8	2,167.5	2,349.7	2,423.5	2,486.8	2,618.4	2,773.8	2,851.0	3,091.8	3,291.3
Under 28 days		1,400.9	1,466.4	1,631.0	1,678.1	1,719.7	1,785.7	1,922.2	1,960.2	2,142.7	2,254.7
Under 1 day		802.7	807.2	921.1	940.2	963.1	1,022.8	1,125.3	1,150.7	1,285.2	1,364.0
1 day		142.9	159.9	177.9	202.3	225.3	226.6	237.5	258.9	286.5	285.7
2 days		108.7	108.6	120.8	128.8	119.8	130.4	140.0	147.3	147.8	150.3
3 days		54.9	55.4	62.8	62.0	67.3	74.4	77.3	74.2	73.9	75.3
4 days		34.5	39.5	40.0	43.9	41.4	41.6	47.8	51.2	52.0	52.6
5 days		28.1	34.0	40.2	37.5	38.3	35.8	29.9	38.8	37.3	37.9
6 days		22.4	23.0	28.5	23.3	28.4	30.9	27.2	24.4	29.3	29.3
7-13 days		96.6	118.5	122.1	118.9	115.7	103.4	109.8	101.4	106.1	124.0
14-20 days		60.6	67.0	67.8	68.7	64.2	63.7	67.0	58.6	64.1	70.9
21-27 days		49.5	53.5	49.8	52.5	56.1	56.0	60.4	54.7	62.5	64.6
28-59 days		177.7	181.7	188.9	200.4	206.1	213.3	215.0	221.1	236.0	256.7
2 months		146.1	144.1	146.0	140.2	154.4	165.7	150.6	171.5	187.0	196.0
3 months		107.6	103.8	108.6	116.3	104.6	119.0	119.8	122.6	133.1	149.4
4 months		74.8	70.8	71.5	80.7	85.8	84.1	96.9	90.8	97.3	111.6
5 months		56.1	53.8	52.8	52.7	57.7	60.2	67.0	71.5	77.5	84.7
6 months		41.4	43.3	41.8	40.5	40.2	47.1	50.4	55.0	55.6	64.1
7 months		27.6	27.7	27.7	33.8	28.9	37.0	39.1	41.8	47.6	46.2
8 months		24.7	25.0	25.3	22.8	24.1	29.5	38.2	35.1	32.5	39.6
9 months		17.8	19.0	23.7	22.8	23.6	23.0	25.5	32.5	29.2	33.0
10 months		17.2	15.4	18.3	16.9	20.0	25.6	25.5	24.0	26.7	25.9
11 months		13.8	16.4	15.8	18.2	21.6	23.0	23.6	24.8	26.4	28.5

*Excludes deaths of U.S. nonresidents
†Deaths based on a 50% sample
*1982 rates rounded in conversion to rate per 100,000
Source: *Vital Statistics of the U.S.*, Vol. II, *Mortality* 1978 Vol. 33 No. 9 Supplement 1984

vironmental factors affect black families more adversely than they do white. Poor nutrition, less knowledgeable child care practices, and scarcer medical care may be chiefly responsible for higher black mortality after these babies leave the hospital. This pattern is prevalent in undeveloped countries as well.

U.S. GEOGRAPHICAL DIFFERENCES

Differences in mortality for infants by race can also be ranked by state (Table 2–5). The New England, Mountain, and Pacific States have the lowest mortality rates for both white and black infants even though the rates differ widely. In the South, where a higher proportion of black infants are born, the overall mortality rate is highest.

The great strides in lowering black infant mortality since 1971 are seen in the East-South-Central states where black infant mortality has been cut by 38.5%. In the Middle Atlantic states, the rate's been cut by 33% and in the Mountain states by 36.3%.

TABLE 2–5.   Infant Mortality Rates (per 1,000 live births) According to Race, Geographic Division, and State: United States, Average Annual 1971–1973, 1976–1978, and 1981–83 (Data are based on the National Vital Statistics System)

GEOGRAPHIC DIVISION AND STATE	All Races			White			Black		
	1971–73*	1976–78*	1981–83	1971–73*	1976–78*	1981–83	1971–73*	1976–78*	1981–83
United States	18.5	14.4	11.6	16.4	12.5	10.1	29.4	24.1	19.6
New England:	16.1	11.9	10.1	15.5	11.3	9.5	27.9	22.6	19.0
Maine	17.6	10.3	9.5	17.7	10.4	9.6	10.0†	9.0†	14.0†
New Hampshire	16.9	10.7	9.8	16.9	10.8	9.8	26.0†	4.0†	19.5†
Vermont	14.8	12.1	8.6	14.9	12.1	8.5	–†	30.3†	28.2†
Massachusetts	15.6	11.7	9.6	15.0	11.2	9.2	28.2	19.6	17.1
Rhode Island	18.6	13.4	11.2	18.1	12.4	10.6	29.9†	30.5	19.3†
Connecticut	15.7	13.1	11.1	14.3	11.5	9.8	27.7	25.1	21.1
Middle Atlantic:	17.7	14.5	11.8	15.6	12.5	10.1	28.8	23.9	19.4
New York	17.7	14.8	12.0	15.6	12.6	10.4	28.0	23.8	18.7
New Jersey	17.7	14.1	11.3	14.7	11.5	9.4	30.4	24.5	19.4
Pennsylvania	17.7	14.4	11.6	16.1	13.0	10.3	29.1	23.8	21.0
East North Central:	18.6	14.4	12.1	16.4	12.6	10.3	31.2	25.2	22.5
Ohio	18.0	14.0	11.7	16.3	12.8	10.3	29.9	22.5	20.3
Indiana	18.6	14.0	11.5	17.3	12.9	10.6	30.6	23.2	19.3
Illinois	20.5	16.1	13.3	17.3	13.0	10.6	32.9	28.2	24.0
Michigan	18.7	14.3	12.4	16.1	12.3	10.1	31.2	24.9	24.2
Wisconsin	14.9	11.7	9.8	14.3	11.2	9.2	24.7	19.2	18.0

GEOGRAPHIC DIVISION AND STATE	All Races			White			Black		
	1971–73*	1976–78*	1981–83	1971–73*	1976–78*	1981–83	1971–73*	1976–78*	1981–83
West North Central:	17.5	13.6	10.6	16.6	12.6	9.9	28.7	25.8	19.3
Minnesota	16.7	12.3	9.9	16.5	12.0	9.5	28.0[†]	24.8[†]	22.1[†]
Iowa	17.0	13.1	9.7	16.9	12.8	9.5	25.2[†]	25.9[†]	20.5[†]
Missouri	18.7	14.8	11.7	16.8	12.7	10.4	29.0	26.6	19.5
North Dakota	15.5	13.6	10.2	15.0	13.1	9.7	30.5[†]	23.7[†]	10.6[†]
South Dakota	18.8	15.6	10.8	16.8	14.0	9.0	33.1[†]	22.2[†]	14.1[†]
Nebraska	17.0	13.3	9.9	16.3	12.8	9.5	31.7[†]	24.1[†]	17.3[†]
Kansas	17.5	13.3	10.7	16.8	12.5	10.2	27.3	24.0	18.0
South Atlantic:	20.2	16.0	13.2	16.8	12.8	10.4	29.2	24.1	20.3
Delaware	16.8	13.2	12.5	13.1	10.7	9.5	31.3	21.9	21.7
Maryland	16.6	15.4	12.1	14.0	12.3	9.4	25.3	23.4	18.7
District of Columbia	27.1	26.6	21.8	20.5	12.9[†]	12.0[†]	28.3	29.5	24.0
Virginia	19.8	15.3	12.4	17.1	12.7	10.3	30.1	24.3	19.6
West Virginia	19.8	15.5	11.8	19.3	15.3	11.6	33.5[†]	23.0[†]	18.6[†]
North Carolina	22.3	16.7	13.3	18.4	13.4	10.7	32.0	24.6	19.8
South Carolina	22.3	18.6	15.7	17.0	13.5	11.9	31.2	26.5	21.8
Georgia	19.9	15.6	13.3	16.3	12.2	9.9	27.6	22.0	19.3
Florida	19.4	14.9	12.8	16.4	12.1	10.1	28.5	23.0	20.8
East South Central:	21.6	16.4	13.1	17.8	13.3	10.7	32.2	24.9	19.8
Kentucky	17.9	13.9	11.9	17.2	13.3	11.4	25.0	21.3	17.8
Tennessee	20.6	15.4	12.5	18.1	13.4	10.3	30.0	22.9	20.2
Alabama	22.7	17.5	13.3	17.7	13.5	10.3	32.6	25.2	19.0
Mississippi	26.3	19.4	15.3	18.6	12.7	10.5	35.0	26.8	20.5
West South Central:	19.9	15.5	11.6	18.0	13.4	10.3	28.2	24.4	17.9
Arkansas	19.3	15.7	10.9	17.3	13.3	9.0	25.3	23.1	16.9
Louisiana	21.6	17.7	13.4	17.9	12.6	9.8	27.6	25.6	19.6
Oklahoma	17.9	14.8	11.7	17.4	14.0	11.5	28.3	22.9	16.7
Texas	19.9	15.0	11.2	18.3	13.5	10.4	29.3	24.0	16.9
Mountain:	17.4	12.8	10.1	16.8	12.4	9.9	25.1	19.4	16.0
Montana	20.7	13.9	9.9	20.1	13.4	9.6	34.2[†]	5.9[†]	29.1[†]
Idaho	16.9	12.0	10.0	16.6	12.1	10.1	20.8[†]	20.1[†]	20.4[†]
Wyoming	22.7	14.4	10.1	22.5	14.4	10.2	40.8[†]	27.2[†]	12.4[†]
Colorado	17.3	12.0	9.7	17.2	11.9	9.7	21.7	19.0	13.1
New Mexico	19.7	14.5	10.4	18.5	13.8	10.2	28.1[†]	23.1[†]	13.5[†]
Arizona	16.9	13.9	10.2	15.7	12.9	9.7	26.0	18.4	17.0
Utah	13.5	11.1	9.9	13.3	10.9	9.9	25.5[†]	19.4[†]	18.5[†]
Nevada	19.4	13.5	10.7	18.7	13.1	10.2	26.2[†]	19.4[†]	19.7[†]
Pacific:	15.9	12.3	10.0	15.3	11.8	9.8	25.1	19.9	16.1
Washington	17.3	13.0	10.2	16.9	12.9	10.0	28.9	18.8	17.0
Oregon	16.7	12.6	10.4	16.6	12.5	10.3	28.0[†]	20.6[†]	16.3[†]
California	15.6	12.1	9.9	14.9	11.5	9.6	24.9	20.0	16.0
Alaska	18.7	15.2	12.0	18.3	13.4	10.4	22.7[†]	20.3[†]	20.9[†]
Hawaii	15.4	11.1	9.3	15.5	11.1	9.6	12.6[†]	12.8[†]	12.2[†]

*Excludes births and infant deaths occurring to U.S. nonresidents.
†States with fewer than 5,000 live births for the 3-year period.
Source: National Center for Health Statistics: Data computed by the Division of Analysis from data compiled by the Division of Vital Statistics.

PERINATAL, NEONATAL, AND POSTNEONATAL MORTALITY RATES

The commonly used infant mortality rate is often broken down into three sub-sets to show infant deaths by general endogenous (internal) or exogenous (external) cause. One sub-set is the neonatal rate. This represents the infants who die within 28 days of birth per 1,000 births. Death is commonly caused by endogenous factors, such as congenital malformations, low birth weight, or birth trauma.

Typically distinct from the neonatal rate is the perinatal rate. It reflects the deaths of both fetuses gestated more than 28 weeks and newborn babies through the first week of life. It includes miscarriages and stillbirths, deaths that are not generally included in the neonatal rate. Some overlap exists, however, between the neo- and perinatal numbers, since both include deaths, due mostly to endogenous factors, during the first week of life.

The third commonly used rate, the postneonatal death rate, reflects those infants dying between age 28 days and 1 year. These deaths are often from exogenous factors, including infectious, parasitic, and respiratory diseases and accidents. Both the U.S. neonatal and general infant mortality rate for the first year of life have been falling (Fig. 2–1). The rate for infants is steeper than that for neonates for most of the last 50 years. Since the infant rate includes neonates, the difference between the two rates is between the postneonatal 28 day to one year rate and the neonatal rate. The steeper decline in the postneonatal rate reflects a safer and healthier environment.

The effect of better environmental conditions is also seen in the difference in the postneonatal rates for different races (Fig. 2–2). During the 1950s and 1960s, the white postneonatal rate fell as environmental factors improved. These factors changed little for black postneonatal infants. By 1965, however, when the socioeconomic status of blacks began to improve, the black postneonatal death rate, although still higher than the white, fell sharply: 4.9%, which exceeded the 3.0% rate of decline for white infants.

Throughout the period, the rate differential is greatest not for the neonatal but for the postneonatal period when environmental factors, particularly the mother's educational level, have the strongest bearing on longevity.

The neonatal death rate for black infants is 80% higher than it is for white infants. But the postneonatal black rate as of the 1970s

FIG. 2–1.   Decline in infant mortality

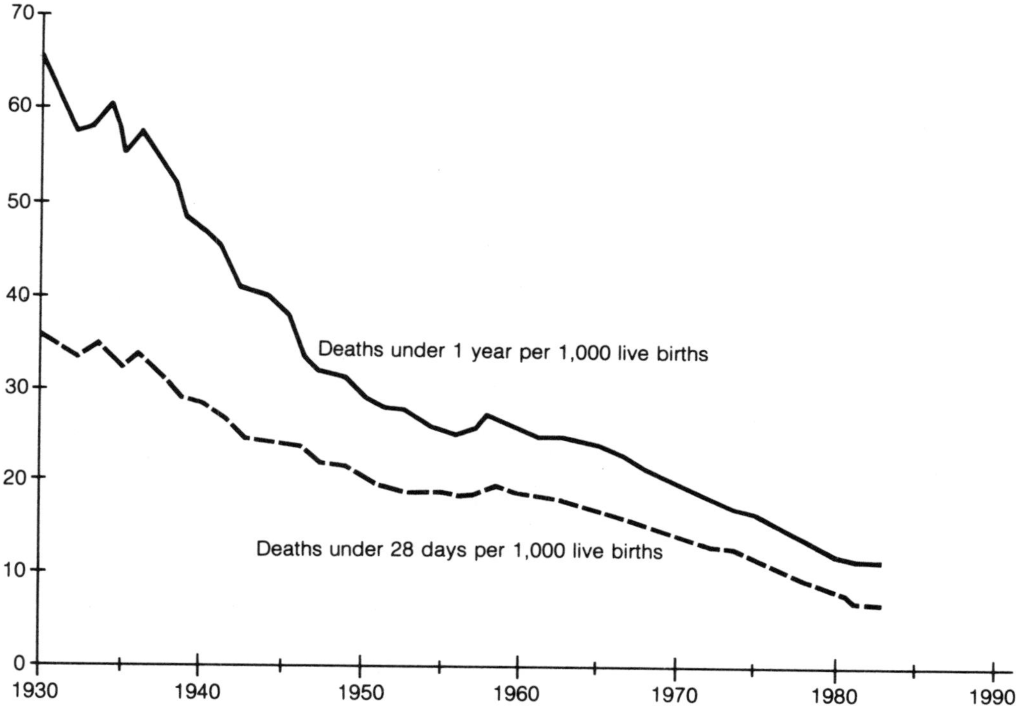

Infant and neonatal mortality rates 1930–1983

Source: *Monthly Vital Statistics Report*, Vol. 32, No. 13, Sept. 1984

was 200% or two times higher than the white rate. For both racial groups, however, the neonatal risk is much higher than the post-neonatal risk; this is characteristic of developed countries. The neonatal rate for both black and white infants reached a plateau, in the 1950s and advances were meager until the late 1960s. Then, the number of low birth weight infants began to drop, and better perinatal units were developed to preserve critically ill or imma-ture infants. The neonatal rate went down dramatically. The neo- and postneonatal death rates for white and black infants are shown in Table 2–6. Other minorities are shown in Table 2–7. The dis-parity in mortality between black and white infants is greatest for the postneonatal period.

Recent U.S. infant mortality rates reflect a drop in deaths from late gestation through birth and from the first to fourth week of life—a decline in the peri- and neonatal death rates. These declines reflect the remarkable technological advances in microsurgery, ge-netic screening, and fetal normalcy testing, including amniocen-

FIG. 2–2.   Neo- and postneonatal mortality rates, according to race: United States, 1950–79.

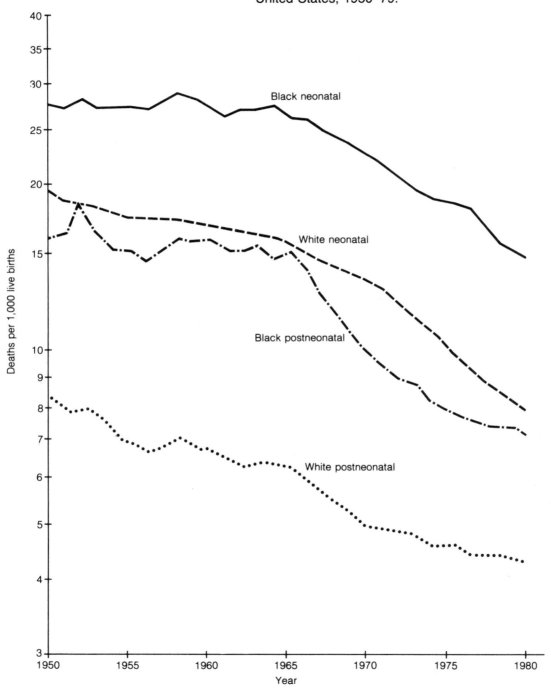

TABLE 2–6.   Infant, Fetal and Perinatal Mortality rates, according to Race: United States Selected years 1950–84 (Data are based on the National Vital Statistics System)

| RACE AND YEAR | INFANT MORTALITY RATE* | | | |
	Total	(Neonatal) Under 28 days	(Neonatal) Under 7 days	Postneonatal
All Races:	Number of deaths per 1,000 live births			
1950	29.2	20.5	17.8	8.7
1960	26.0	18.7	16.7	7.3
1970	20.0	15.1	13.6	4.9
1975	16.1	11.6	10.0	4.5
1976	15.2	10.9	9.3	4.3
1977	14.1	9.9	8.4	4.2
1978	13.8	9.5	8.0	4.3
1979	13.1	8.9	7.5	4.2
1980	12.6	8.5	7.1	4.1
1981	11.9	8.0	6.7	3.9
1982	11.5	7.7	6.4	3.8
1983	11.2	7.3	6.1	3.9
1984	10.6	6.9	—	3.7
White:				
1950	26.8	19.4	17.1	7.4
1960	22.9	17.2	15.6	5.7
1970	17.8	13.8	12.5	4.0
1975	14.2	10.4	9.0	3.8
1976	13.3	9.7	8.2	3.6
1977	12.3	8.7	7.4	3.6
1978	12.0	8.4	7.0	3.6
1979	11.4	7.9	6.6	3.5
1980	11.0	7.5	6.2	3.5
1981	10.5	7.1	5.9	3.4
1982	10.1	6.8	5.6	3.3
1983	9.7	6.4	5.4	3.3
Black:				
1950	43.9	27.8	23.0	16.1
1960	44.3	27.8	23.7	16.5
1970	32.6	22.8	20.3	9.9
1975	26.2	18.3	15.7	7.9
1976	25.5	17.9	15.3	7.6
1977	23.6	16.1	13.5	7.6
1978	23.1	15.5	13.2	7.6
1979	21.8	14.3	12.1	7.5
1980	21.4	14.1	11.9	7.3
1981	20.0	13.4	11.4	6.6
1982	19.6	13.1	11.1	6.6
1983	19.2	12.4	10.6	6.8

*Infant mortality rate is the number of deaths of infants under 1 year of age per 1,000 live births. Neonatal deaths occur within 28 days of birth; postneonatal deaths occur from 28 days to 365 days after birth. Deaths within 7 days are considered early neonatal deaths.
Sources: National Center for Health Statistics: *Vital Statistics of the United States*, Vol. II, Mortality, Part A, 1950–83. Public Health Service. Washington, U.S. Government Printing Office: Annual summary of births, deaths, marriages, and divorces, United States, 1984. *Monthly Vital Statistics Report*. Vol. 33–No. 13. DHHS Pub. No. (PHS) 84-1120. Public Health Service. Hyattsville, Md., Sept. 26, 1985; Data computed by the Division of Analysis from data compiled by the Division of Vital Statistics.

TABLE 2–7.   Neo- and Postneonatal Mortality rates (deaths per 1,000 live births) According to Race, United States, Selected Years, 1950–77

YEAR	Black	American Indian	Chinese-American	Japanese-American	White
Neonatal mortality rate*					
1970	22.8	10.6	5.4	8.4	13.8
1977	16.1	8.3	4.2	5.1	8.7
Postneonatal mortality rate[†]					
1970[‡]	9.9	11.4	3.1	2.2	4.0
1977[‡]	7.6	7.3	1.7	1.5	3.6

*Deaths of infants within 28 days of birth per 1,000 live births.
[†]Deaths of infants 28 to 365 days old per 1,000 live births.
[‡]Excludes deaths of nonresidents of the United States.
Source: Division of Vital Statistics, National Center for Health Statistics: selected data.

tesis and critical intensive care available for very low birth weight babies that could not have survived out of the womb until a few years ago.

Within the last decade, several advanced technology perinatal units have been established at hospitals throughout the country. These facilities play a significant role in caring for critically ill and low birth rate babies and increasing their survival rates. The costs, however, are substantial. The March of Dimes noted an average cost of $28,884 for infants weighing 1,000 g or less studied at Babies Hospital in New York City in 1980. The average cost for 91 infants in the study who weighed between 2,001 and 2,500 g was $8,487.

TABLE 2–8.   Infant Weight-specific Mortality Rates*

WEIGHT IN GRAMS (POUNDS)	New Mexico (1974–1977)	New York (1968)	United States (1960)
⩽ 1,000 (⩽ 2.25)	801.1	847.2	919.3[†]
1,001–1,500 (2.26–3.29)	340.1	379.5	548.5[†]
1,501–2,000 (3.30–4.39)	119.9	131.1	206.6[†]
2,001–2,500 (4.40–5.50)	30.2	34.9	58.4[†]
> 2,500 (> 5.50)	7.0	8.4[‡]	11.2[†]
Unknown	855.9	132.3[‡]	—
Total**	16.4	21.9[‡]	25.1[†]

*Number of individuals who died before 365 days of age per 1,000 live births
[†]Significantly different, at the 95% level, from New York's and New Mexico's rates
[‡]Significantly different, at the 95% level, from New Mexico's rates
**Data for all weight categories combined (including unknown)
Source: *Morbidity and Mortality Weekly Report*, Vol. 32, No. 8, Mar. 1983

TABLE 2–9.   U.S. Fetal and Perinatal Death Rate, 1950–83

YEAR	INFANT MORTALITY RATE*		
	Fetal death rate[†]	Late fetal death rate[‡]	Perinatal mortality rate**
All Races:			
1950[¶]	18.4	14.9	32.5
1960[¶]	15.8	12.1	28.6
1970	14.0	9.5	23.0
1975	10.6	7.8	17.7
1976	10.3	7.5	16.7
1977	9.8	7.1	15.4
1978	9.6	6.6	14.6
1979	9.3	6.4	13.8
1980	9.1[‖]	6.2[‖]	13.2[‖]
1981	8.9	5.9	12.6
1982	8.8	5.9	12.3
1983	8.4	5.4	11.5
1984[¶,§]	—	—	—
Whites:			
1950[¶]	16.6	13.3	30.1
1960[¶]	13.9	10.8	26.2
1970	12.3	8.6	21.1
1975	9.4	7.1	16.0
1976	9.3	6.9	15.1
1977	8.7	6.5	13.9
1978	8.4	6.0	13.0
1979	8.3	5.9	12.5
1980	8.1[‖]	5.7[‖]	11.9[‖]
1981	8.0	5.5	11.3
1982	7.9	5.5	11.0
1983	7.4	5.0	10.3
Blacks:			
1950[¶]	32.1	—	—
1960[¶]	—	—	—
1970	23.2	—	—
1975	16.8	11.4	26.9
1976	16.0	10.7	25.8
1977	15.6	10.1	23.5
1978	15.6	9.7	22.7
1979	14.8	9.0	21.1
1980	14.4[‖]	8.9[‖]	20.7[‖]
1981	13.8	8.2	19.4
1982	13.8	8.2	19.1
1983	13.5	7.7	18.2

*Infant mortality rate is the number of deaths of infants under 1 year of age per 1,000 live births, neonatal deaths occur within 28 days of birth; postneonatal deaths occur from 28 days to 365 days after birth, deaths within 7 days are considered early neonatal deaths.
[†]Number of deaths of fetuses of 20 weeks or more gestation per 1,000 live births plus fetal deaths.
[‡]Number of fetal deaths of 28 weeks or more gestation per 1,000 live births plus late fetal deaths.
**Number of late fetal deaths plus infant deaths within 7 days of birth per 1,000 live births plus late fetal deaths.
[¶]Includes births and infant and late fetal deaths occurring to United States nonresidents
[‖]Revised figures
[§]Provisional data, not available separately by race
Sources: National Center for Health Statistics: *Vital Statistics of the United States*, Vol. II, Mortality, Part A, 1950–83. Public Health Service. Washington, U.S. Government Printing Office; Annual summary of births, deaths, marriages, and divorces, United States, 1984. *Monthly Vital Statistics Report*. Vol. 33-No. 13. DHHS Pub. No. (PHS) 84-1120. Public Health Service. Hyattsville, Md., Sept. 26, 1985; Data computed by the Division of Analysis from data compiled by the Division of Vital Statistics.

Table 2–8 summarizes the mortality rates in New Mexico, New York City, and the United States for low birth weight infants at specific weight intervals. The rising number of abortions occurring at a higher rate among high-risk than among low-risk pregnancies also helps reduce these rates. The perinatal death rates in the United States from 1950 to 1983 are shown in Table 2–9.

The 1978 U.S. perinatal death rate of 14.6 (15.2 when computed for international comparison to include fetal deaths of unknown gestation) was not the lowest rate compared to other industrialized nations. Table 2–10 shows that several countries have reduced perinatal mortality more in recent years. Austria, Denmark, the German Federal Republic, Sweden, and Switzerland have all had slightly greater reductions than the United States. By 1978, Sweden and Switzerland, reported rates roughly 30% lower than the United States. However, the population in these countries is not as socioeconomically heterogeneous as that in the United States.

In Chapter 3 discussion of the causes of infant mortality will reveal the reasons for some of these differences in perinatal death rates.

TABLE 2–10.   International Perinatal Death Rate

COUNTRY	PERINATAL MORTALITY RATIO*		Average Annual Change 1973–78 (%)
	1973[†]	1978[‡]	
	Perinatal deaths (per 1,000 live births)		
Canada**	17.7	15.1	−5.2
United States	20.7	15.2	−6.0
Austria	24.8	15.0	−9.6
Denmark**	14.6	10.7	−7.5
England and Wales	21.3	17.1	−5.3
France**	18.8	15.8	−3.4
German Dem Republic	19.4	15.2	−4.8
German Fed Republic	23.2	13.8	−9.9
Ireland**	23.1	21.8	−2.9
Italy	29.6	20.8	−6.8
Netherlands**	16.4	13.0	−5.6
Sweden	14.1	9.6	−7.3
Switzerland	15.5	10.7	−7.1
Israel	21.2	17.4	−3.9
Japan	18.0	13.0	−6.3
Australia**	22.4	17.8	−5.6
New Zealand**	19.4	14.3	−5.0

*Fetal deaths of 28 weeks or more gestation plus infant deaths within 7 days per 1,000 live births. For all countries, fetal deaths of unknown gestation period are included in the 28 weeks or more gestation. This is not the usual way of calculating the perinatal ratio for the United States, but it was done for the purpose of comparison.
[†]Data for New Zealand refer to 1971; data for France, German Democratic Republic, and Italy refer to 1972.
[‡]Data for Ireland refer to 1975; data for Canada, Denmark, England and Wales, France, German Democratic Republic, Italy, Netherlands, Australia, and New Zealand refer to 1977; data for France are provisional.
**Data for Canada, Ireland, Italy, Australia, and New Zealand refer to 1977; data for Denmark and France are provisional.
Sources: World Health Organization: World Health Statistics, 1973–76 and 1980. Vol. 1, Geneva. World Health Organization, 1976 and 1980; United Nations: *Demographic Yearbook 1974*. Pub. No. St/ESA/STAT/R.3. New York, United Nations, 1975.

Causes of Infant Mortality and Morbidity 3

The overall U.S. neonatal death rate is roughly twice as high as the postneonatal rate. The individual rates for neonatal conditions, such as congenital anomalies, low birth weight, birth trauma, respiratory distress syndrome, and other perinatal conditions all have higher rates than those for postneonatal causes such as certain gastrointestinal diseases. Table 3–1 shows the death rates for the 10 leading causes of infant death including endogenous and exogenous causes for 1983 and 1984.

NEONATAL MORTALITY

CONGENITAL ANOMALIES

In 1984, 8,180 deaths in the United States resulted from congenital anomalies. In fact, congenital anomalies are the leading cause of infant mortality and morbidity. Birth defects, as congenital anomalies are commonly called, can be either structural or functional or both and may involve any of the body's major systems. Spina bifida, e.g., one of the more frequent defects, in which the spine is exposed at the surface of the body, is a central nervous system (CNS) anomaly.

TABLE 3–1.   Death under 1 Year in the Sample and Estimated Infant Mortality Rates, by Age and for 10 Selected Causes: United States, 12 Months Ending with August 1983 and 1984 (rates on an annual basis per 1,000 live births adjusted for changing numbers of births)

AGE AND CAUSE OF DEATH (NINTH REVISION INTERNATIONAL CLASSIFICATION OF DISEASES, 1975)		12 MONTHS ENDING WITH AUGUST			
		1984 (Number	Rate)	1983 (Number	Rate)
Total, under 1 year		3,924	10.7	4,072	11.0
Under 28 days		2,535	6.9	2,732	7.4
28 days to 11 months		1,389	3.8	1,340	3.6
Certain gastrointestinal diseases	008-009,535,555-558	32	0.1	26	0.1
Pneumonia and influenza	480-487	61	0.2	76	0.2
Congenital anomalies	740-759	818	2.2	855	2.3
Disorders relating to short gestation and unspecified low birth weight	765	331	0.9	350	0.9
Birth trauma	767	35	0.1	49	0.1
Intrauterine hypoxia and birth asphyxia	768	110	0.3	124	0.3
Respiratory distress syndrome	769	390	1.1	370	1.0
Other conditions originating in the perinatal period	760-764,766,770-779	1,001	2.7	1,061	2.9
Sudden infant death syndrome	798.0	514	1.4	491	1.3
All other causes	Residual	632	1.7	670	1.8

Source: *Monthly Vital Statistics Report*, Vol. 33, No. 9 Dec. 1984

Another common defect is a hole between the lower chambers of the heart, called ventricular septal defect. Cleft lip and cleft palate, in which the two sides of the face fail to join at the lip or palate, are also common. They are classified as defects of the alimentary system. Genitourinary system defects include undescended testicles and cystic kidney disease.

Several different defects affect limb formation, such as club foot, in which the foot turns outward; polydactyly, the formation of extra fingers or toes; and reduction deformities, in which limbs are incompletely developed. A common metabolic disorder is an amino acid deficiency called phenylketonuria (PKU). A defect like Down's syndrome, however, is a multisystem one because it alters physical appearance and causes mental retardation.

The International Clearinghouse for Birth Defects Monitoring Systems has selected 11 congenital conditions for international comparison on a regular quarterly basis. These conditions are easily recognizable at birth, defined consistently across medical communities around the world, occur often enough to permit reliable calculation of their rates, and may be environmentally caused.

Monitoring programs vary from country to country. Some programs obtain data from hospitals, others directly from population groups (Table 3–2). Because of variations in the numbers of births observed and the exclusion of stillbirths in the data denominator of three participating programs (Mexico, South America, and Spain),

TABLE 3–2.   Birth Defects per 10,000 Live Births in Reporting Countries for 1981

MONITORING PROGRAMS	Anencephaly	Hydrocephaly	Cleft Lip	Anorectal Atresia	Reduction Deformity	Down's Syndrome	Cleft Palate	Esophageal Atresia	Hypospadias
Canada	4.7	2.7	9.0	1.7	3.4	—	3.8	1.0	12.9
Czechoslovakia	3.5	2.9	11.3	2.8	5.2	8.7	7.4	1.9	19.9
Denmark	2.4	1.9	13.7	0.9	6.2		3.6	0.9	12.6
England/Wales	3.9	2.9	9.5	2.5	4.0	7.3	4.1	1.8	15.9
Finland	2.2	2.8	5.8	0.9	4.9	NA	11.3	1.9	5.2
France	1.2	1.3	6.0	1.2	4.2	13.0	1.4	1.3	4.3
Hungary	6.0	4.7	13.7	4.4	4.4		5.6	5.2	24.3
Israel	6.7	2.2	4.5	5.6	6.7		3.4	2.2	31.4
Italy	3.7	3.1	8.4	4.9	8.2	13.9	4.9	3.1	1.9
Japan	5.2	1.6	10.0	2.1	5.8	6.7	3.1	1.0	2.1
Mexico	3.9	4.7	7.8	1.4	6.1		2.5	0.6	2.2
New Zealand	2.8	4.0	7.6	2.2	3.8	8.2	5.4	0.8	9.8
Northern Ireland	17.4	4.7	10.9	8.0	7.6	17.2	9.4	4.7	8.4
Norway	4.5	3.5	15.1	2.2	8.4	9.9	4.1	1.8	11.6
South America	4.0	4.0	11.3	4.0	6.8		3.1	2.6	8.0
Spain	3.1	2.9	7.2	2.4	8.9	15.4	4.9	1.7	17.1
Sweden	1.2	4.2	15.4	4.5	6.6	12.9	6.5	3.6	19.9
USA-Atlanta	3.0	9.7	10.4	3.7	14.1	9.5	2.6	4.5	25.0

Source: International Clearinghouse for Birth Defects Monitoring Systems, Annual Report, 1981

the data should be reviewed with caution. U.S. data come from the Atlanta Disease Control Centers' population-based metropolitan Atlanta Monitoring Program.

The monitored conditions which can be grouped by body systems comprise:

The Brain and Head:
Anencephaly—absence of roof of skull and part or all of brain
Spina bifida—incompletely closed spine with herniation of the spinal cord
Hydrocephaly—enlarged head due to obstruction of cerebrospinal fluid flow
Cleft palate—unfused palate
Cleft lip—unfused lip

Digestive System:
Esophageal atresia or stenosis—closure or narrowing of the esophagus with or without an opening to the trachea
Anorectal atresia or stenosis—absence of anus or narrowing of anal canal
Hypospadias—abnormal opening of male urethra on underside of penis

Limbs:

Reduction deformity—absence or atrophied limbs or parts thereof

Multi-system Condition:

Down's syndrome—retardation

The incidence of these same conditions for the United States by geographic region in 1982 is listed in Table 3–3. These data were gathered by the Atlanta Centers' national monitoring program.[a]

Difficulties in collecting data are perhaps best illustrated by the fact that the incidence of congenital anomalies at birth is higher among black babies than among white. But follow-up studies show no racial difference in the number of anomalies accumulated by age 5 years. On follow-up, severe defects showed a 4% incidence, whereas moderate ones showed an 11% incidence. The rates were highest for children who weighed 2500 or less at birth.[b]

The Birth Defects Monitoring Program of the Centers for Disease Control recently compared the rates of the most common birth defects. The information was from hospital records collected by the Commission on Professional and Hospital Activities in the early 1970s compared with those collected in the early 1980s. During this period, more than 13 million births at 1,000 participating hospitals were reviewed. Defects were grouped as to whether their incidence rates rose by 2% or more, stayed within 2% of their 1970s rate, or fell by 2% or more since the early 1970s.

Tables 3–4, 3–5, and 3–6 summarize the results for conditions that rose, fell, and remained about the same. Conditions with a higher incidence included ventricular septal defects, patent ductus arteriosus, coarctation of the aorta, and valvular stenosis and atresia. Although reasons for the rise are unknown, analysts surmise that more detailed diagnoses during the intervals shown when surgical repairs became possible, led to higher incidence reports. Lower parity rates and improved postpartum treatment for women with Rh factor problems led to a fall in the rate of Rh hemolytic newborn disease during the same period. For unknown reasons, rates of spina bifida and anencephaly also fell.

The causes of neonatal congenital defects are largely unknown. They may range from genetic defects passed from the parents gene

[a]The accuracy of these data is questionable in view of the discrepancy between hydrospadias incidence figures reported for each section of the country gathered by Atlanta's national monitoring program and the national figure gathered by Atlanta's local monitoring program (Table 3–3) and reported internationally. The national figure is much lower than any of the area numbers.

[b]Christianson MA, Von Den Berg MD, Milkovich, et al: Frank incidence of congenital anomalies among white and black live births with long-term follow-up. *Public Health* 71:12, pp 1333–1340, Dec 1981

TABLE 3–3. U.S. Congenital Malformations, 1980*

CONDITION	Northeast	North Central	South	West	Total
Anencephaly	3.7	3.1	3.8	2.5	3.3
Hydrocephaly	3.9	3.9	4.6	3.4	4.0
Cleft lip	6.6	8.4	7.7	8.9	8.0
Reduction deformity	4.4	3.9	3.4	3.8	3.8
Rectal atresia	4.1	3.6	3.2	2.6	3.4
Down's syndrome	8.9	7.4	5.7	8.6	7.3
Cleft palate	3.9	5.2	4.6	5.4	4.9
Spina bifida	3.8	5.1	6.9	4.0	5.2
Tracheo/Esophageal Fistula	1.9	2.2	1.7	1.9	2.0
Hypospadias	58.7	53.8	45.6	44.8	50.8

*Incidence rate per 10,000 live births
Source: Atlanta Center for Disease Control Congential Malfunctions Surveillance

TABLE 3–4. Malformations with Increased Rates, Birth Defects Monitoring Program, United States, 1970–1971 and 1982–1983

MALFORMATION	Cases		Rates*		Mean Annual Change (%)
	1970–1971	1982–1983	1970–1971	1982–1983	
Congenital cataract	110	153	0.64	0.97	+3.5
Tetralogy of Fallot	99	145	0.57	0.92	+4.4
Ventricular septal defect	770	2,411	4.45	15.23	+10.8
Valve stenosis and atresia	217	434	1.25	2.74	+6.8
Patent ductus arteriosus	686	4,355	3.96	7.50	+17.5
Coarctation of aorta	72	95	0.42	0.60	+3.0
Congenital ureteral obstruction	187	301	1.08	1.90	+4.8
Hypospadias	3,565	4,471	20.60	28.23	+2.7
Renal agenesis	123	278	0.71	1.76	+7.9
Congenital hip dislocation without CNS defects	1,382	4,579	7.99	8.92	+11.3
Autosomal abnormality excluding Down's syndrome	197	322	1.14	2.03	+4.9

*Cases per 10,000 total births.
Source: *Morbidity and Mortality Weekly Report*, Vol. 34, No. 2SS

TABLE 3–5. Malformations with Decreased Rates, Birth Defects Monitoring Program, United States, 1970–1971 and 1982–1983

MALFORMATION	Cases		Rates*		Mean Annual Change (%)
	1970–1971	1982–1983	1970–1971	1982–1983	
Anencephaly	949	498	5.48	3.14	−4.5
Spina bifida without anencephaly	1,306	757	7.55	4.78	−3.7
Anophthalmos	74	38	0.43	0.24	−4.7
Congenital rubella	62	28	0.36	0.18	−5.6
Rh-hemolytic newborn disease	7,315	2,474	42.28	15.62	−8.0

*Cases per 10,000 total births.
Source: *Morbidity and Mortality Weekly Report*, Vol. 34, No. 2SS

TABLE 3–6.   Malformations with Stable Rates, Birth Defects Monitoring Program, United States, 1970–1971, and 1982–1983

MALFORMATION	Cases		Rates*		Mean Annual Change (%)
	1970–1971	1982–1983	1970–1971	1982–1983	
Hydrocephalus without spina bifida	833	896	4.81	5.66	1.4
Encephalocele	208	178	1.20	1.12	−0.5
Total CNS	3,803	3,001	21.98	18.95	−1.1
Microphthalmos	94	96	0.54	0.61	+1.0
Aorta pulmonary defect persistent truncus	49	36	0.28	0.23	−1.4
Atrial septal defect	331	269	1.91	1.70	−0.9
Transposition of great arteries	131	149	0.76	0.94	+1.8
Cleft palate without cleft lip	873	820	5.05	5.18	+0.2
Cleft palate with cleft lip	1,073	925	6.20	5.84	−0.5
Cleft lip with or without cleft palate	1,715	1,433	9.91	9.05	−0.7
Tracheoesophageal fistula	289	284	1.67	1.79	−0.6
Rectal atresia and stenosis	648	502	3.75	3.17	−1.2
Cystic kidney disease	200	206	1.16	1.30	+1.0
Bladder extrophy	60	46	0.35	0.29	−1.3
Clubfoot without CNS defects	4,756	4,055	27.49	25.61	−0.6
Reduction deformity	547	584	3.16	3.69	+1.3
Down's syndrome	1,413	1,279	8.17	8.08	−0.01

*Cases per 10,000 total births
Source: Morbidity and Mortality Weekly Report, Vol. 34, No. 2SS

pool to such environmental factors as smoking, excessive alcohol intake during pregnancy, rubella virus, dietary deficiencies, X-ray exposure, and drugs like thalidomide. Pregnant women are thus advised to stay away from children with measles and minimize ingesting drugs, smoking, and drinking alcohol in substantial amounts. They are encouraged to supplement their diet with vitamins and minerals, including calcium. These measures, although not guaranteeing a healthy, well-formed baby, strengthen the odds.

In 1984, the March of Dimes Foundation estimated that more than 30% of the patients in pediatric wards were being treated for congenital defects. Table 3–7 summarizes the hospital days spent by children younger than age 15 years in non-Federal, short-stay hospitals in 1979 and 1981 because of a congenital defect. As indicated, the days increase as more genetically afflicted infants grow into childhood. Although the length of stay is about the same for male and female children, more males than females are hospitalized for congenital anomalies. This fact is reflected in the difference in the days hospitalized in 1981: 716,000 days for males compared to 358,000 for females.

GENETIC DISEASES

Another cause of infant and early childhood mortality and morbidity is congenital disease transmitted through parental genes.

For example, Tay-Sachs disease or sickle-cell anemia are almost always fatal, whereas others, such as hemophilia and PKU are usually chronic conditions.

Tay-Sachs disease, caused by an inborn enzyme deficiency, is common among Jews from eastern and central Europe. It is characterized by loss of muscle tone and motor ability usually within the first year of life. Retardation, blindness, and convulsions follow and death almost always ensues by age five years. Though a rare disease, one in every 30 Jews of Ashkenazic descent carries the Tay-Sachs recessive gene. It causes the disease in 25% of babies whose parents are both carriers. About 1 in 3,600 live births of Ashkenazic Jews develops the disease. Less than an estimated 100 babies are affected in the United States yearly.

Sickle-cell anemia, a congenital hemolytic anemia, occurs in 0.3% of all American blacks. Although not exclusive to blacks, about 12% carry at least one gene for the disease. As the name suggests, the red blood cells (RBCs) are sickle shaped, and cannot travel through the arterioles and capillaries of the circulatory system. This can lead to blood clots and tissue damage due to insufficient oxygen supply. Symptoms include anemia, painful joints, and ulceration of the legs. Survival past age 40 years is unusual. In fact, 50% of victims die earlier than age 25 years.

TABLE 3–7. Days in Non-Federal Short-stay Hospitals for Congential Defects in Patients Younger than Age 15 Years (Data are based on a sample of hospital records)

SEX	Discharges*		Days of Care*		Average Stay[†]	
	1979	1981	1979	1981	1979	1981
Male:	98	118	564	716	5.7	6.1
Total[‡]	1,588	1,632	6,757	7,659	5.3	4.7
Female:	62	72	322	358	5.2	5.0
Total[‡]	2,053	2,101	9,008	9,611	4.4	4.6

*In thousands
[†]In days
[‡]Includes all diagnoses.
Note: Diagnostic categories are based on the *International Classification of Diseases, 9th Revision, Clinical Modification.*
Source: Division of Health Care Statistics, National Center for Health Statistics: Data from the National Hospital Discharge Survey.

Cystic fibrosis is primarily a disorder of northern Europeans. It's the most common fatal genetic disease among Caucasians. In non-Caucasians, it occurs in 1 in 17,000 live births. But in Caucasians, its incidence is 1 in 2,000 live births. It affects the pancreas, respiratory system, and sweat glands. The latter secrete abnormally high levels of substances called electrolytes. The disorder is fatal in 50 percent of patients by age 16 years. Researchers believe it is caused by a biochemical alteration in a protein or enzyme.

If unchecked at birth, phenylketonuria (PKU), another genetic disease, can cause irreversible brain damage and retardation by age 2 years in patients who lack the enzyme for metabolizing phenylalanine, an amino acid essential for growth in children. This disorder can be tested for within 48 hours of birth, and PKU testing is required in most states. One in every 19,000 live births has PKU, and one in 60 persons is an asymptomatic carrier although the ratio is drastically lower for Finns, blacks, and Ashkenazic Jews. If PKU babies are diagnosed early, brain damage can be prevented by putting them on a special nonprotein or low phenylalanine diet.

Other genetic diseases, such as Huntington's chorea can strike fatally as late as middle age. But genetic defects, such as color blindness, are typically non life-threatening.

The March of Dimes Foundation estimates that nearly 200 genetic disorders can be detected before delivery by amniocentesis. This procedure became available in the United States in the 1970s. A needle is inserted through the mother's abdominal wall into the uterus to obtain amniotic fluid. The sample can then be cultured and examined for chromosomal abnormalities and other fetal abnormalities. Although the procedure is not without risk, it's often recommended for pregnant women older than age 35 years who are at greater risk of having an abnormal child. Since Down's syndrome occurs in 1 of every 40 births to women older than age 44 years and to 1 in 280 women over 35 years compared to 1 of 2,500 women younger than 20 years, amniocentesis is a particularly useful screening procedure for this disorder. Data on amniocentesis, gathered by the National Natality Survey in 1980 are shown in Table 3–8.

At present, screening and genetic counseling of prospective parents are the main methods of preventing these diseases. Indeed, despite efforts to treat afflicted children, the greatest hope lies in

TABLE 3–8.   Pregnant Women Receiving Amniocentesis, According to Age, Race, and Residence: United States, 1980

RESIDENCE	< 35 Years (%)			≥ 35 Years (%)		
	All races	White	Black	All races	White	Black
All locations	3.9	3.8	5.0	29.0	30.0	16.7
Metropolitan	4.0	3.7	5.4	33.0	34.8	★
South	4.1	4.5	3.3	23.5	20.6	★
Other regions	3.9	3.5	6.8	35.7	38.5	★
Nonmetropolitan	3.8	3.8	4.0	22.0	22.0	★
South	3.5	3.6	3.6	18.5	19.5	★
Other regions	4.1	3.9	★	25.0	24.0	★

Note: Based on 4,893 births with responses to the item on amniocentesis on the hospital or physician questionnaire
Source: National Center for Health Statistics: Preliminary data from the National Natality Survey

research aimed at preventing genetic diseases and congenital birth defects. With an eye toward prevention, researchers have isolated the factor most often associated with birth defects—low birth weight.

LOW BIRTH WEIGHT

A low birth weight infant is one who weighs less than 5½ pounds or 2,500 g at birth. Since 1935 this has been the accepted definition for the American Academy of Pediatrics. Since 1948, it has been the definition, as well, of the World Health Organization in its Sixth Revision of the International List of Diseases and Causes of Death. Low birth weight infants are either premature or full-term babies who are born small.

According to reports of the Division of Vital Statistics of the Center For Health Statistics, low birth weight babies account for more than one-half of all deaths under 1 year and nearly three-fourths of deaths in the first 28 days of life (neonatal deaths).

From birth certificate information gathered from a majority of the states since 1950, epidemiologists note an increased incidence of low weight births from 1950 to the mid-1960s, from 7.5% to 8.3%. From the mid-1960s through the late-1970s, a decline occurred. It's one of the reasons for the general decline in infant mortality and more specifically in perinatal mortality during the same period. Yet, while the incidence has dropped for all infants, among non-white babies it is still substantially higher than it is for whites.

Table 3–9 shows the dispersion of low birth weight babies by race and geographic regions in the United States. The data as a whole show a slight decline in low birth weight babies for each race from the first period of 1971–1973 to the most recent one, 1981 to 1983. Interestingly, the non-white low birth weight babies in the 1981 to 1983 interval were slightly fewer in the East South Central states than in some of the more affluent states, such as Connecticut, New Jersey, Pennsylvania, Ohio, Illinois, and Michigan. The highest number among blacks occurred in Wyoming.

One possible explanation is that states with traditionally high black populations have made some effort to stress prenatal care, whereas states with few blacks, such as Wyoming, may have no special educational programs for them. Urban blacks also receive less care than do rural blacks in states with large black populations. So states like Illinois and Michigan report a higher rate of low birth weight black babies than do states like Mississippi. Proportionately more black than white infants have a low birth weight, and therefore higher mortality. But differences between their weight

TABLE 3–9. Infants Weighing 2500 g or Less at Birth,* According to Race, Geographic Division, and State: United States (Data are based on the National Vital Statistics System)

GEOGRAPHIC DIVISION AND STATE	All Races			White			Black		
	1971–73	1976–78	1981–83†	1971–73	1976–78	1981–83†	1971–73	1976–78	1981–83†
United States	7.6	7.1	6.8	6.5	6.0	5.7	13.4	12.9	12.5
New England:	7.1	6.4	6.0	6.7	6.0	5.5	13.4	12.5	12.1
Maine	6.4	5.6	5.3	6.4	5.5	5.3	5.5‡	6.8‡	6.0‡
New Hampshire	6.8	5.9	5.1	6.7	5.9	5.1	8.9‡	6.0‡	5.5‡
Vermont	7.0	6.5	6.0	7.0	6.4	6.0	3.3‡	15.4‡	8.5‡
Massachusetts	7.1	6.4	5.9	6.7	6.1	5.5	13.3	11.4	11.1
Rhode Island	7.1	6.7	6.1	6.6	6.2	5.6	14.5‡	13.4‡	11.5‡
Connecticut	7.3	6.9	6.7	6.6	6.0	5.7	13.4	13.6	13.5
Middle Atlantic:	8.0	7.5	7.0	6.7	6.2	5.7	14.1	13.4	12.6
New York	8.2	7.9	7.3	6.9	6.5	5.9	13.9	13.2	12.1
New Jersey	8.0	7.5	7.1	6.5	6.0	5.5	14.4	13.5	13.0
Pennsylvania	7.6	7.0	6.6	6.6	6.0	5.5	14.4	13.7	13.5
East North Central:	7.4	7.0	6.7	6.3	5.8	5.5	13.8	13.4	13.4
Ohio	7.4	6.9	6.7	6.4	5.9	5.7	13.7	13.2	12.9
Indiana	6.8	6.5	6.3	6.2	5.8	5.7	12.0	12.0	12.0
Illinois	7.9	7.5	7.3	6.2	5.8	5.4	14.0	13.7	13.9
Michigan	7.8	7.3	6.9	6.3	6.0	5.6	14.4	13.6	13.7
Wisconsin	6.2	5.6	5.2	5.8	5.2	4.7	12.8	12.4	12.5
West North Central:	6.5	6.0	5.7	6.0	5.5	5.1	13.0	13.0	12.3
Minnesota	5.9	5.3	5.1	5.7	5.2	4.9	12.9‡	11.8‡	11.5‡
Iowa	6.1	5.5	4.9	5.9	5.4	4.8	13.3‡	11.3‡	10.9‡
Missouri	7.4	7.1	6.7	6.3	5.9	5.6	13.3	13.5	12.8
North Dakota	5.8	5.2	4.7	5.6	5.0	4.6	*9.2‡	12.5‡	6.3‡
South Dakota	6.0	5.4	5.2	5.8	5.2	4.8	13.9‡	10.6‡	10.6‡
Nebraska	6.4	5.8	5.5	6.1	5.4	5.0	12.5‡	12.4‡	12.3‡
Kansas	6.6	6.4	6.2	6.1	5.9	5.6	12.1	12.7	12.1
South Atlantic:	8.5	8.1	7.9	6.7	6.2	5.9	13.3	12.8	12.5
Delaware	7.9	7.8	7.4	6.2	6.0	5.5	14.1	13.8	13.4
Maryland	7.9	7.9	7.6	6.2	5.8	5.6	13.0	13.0	12.3
District of Columbia	12.8	12.8	13.3	6.7	7.0‡	6.1‡	13.8	14.0	14.9
Virginia	8.0	7.4	7.2	6.6	5.9	5.7	13.1	12.2	12.1
West Virginia	7.4	6.9	6.8	7.2	6.8	6.7	12.2‡	11.5‡	10.9‡
North Carolina	8.8	8.1	7.9	6.9	6.2	6.0	13.4	12.5	12.3
South Carolina	8.8	8.9	8.8	6.5	6.1	6.2	12.6	13.1	12.8
Georgia	9.3	8.7	8.5	7.0	6.3	6.0	13.8	13.0	12.7
Florida	8.3	7.9	7.4	6.6	6.2	5.9	13.1	12.5	11.9
East South Central:	8.4	8.0	7.9	6.7	6.4	6.2	12.7	12.3	12.2
Kentucky	7.5	7.1	7.0	7.0	6.5	6.5	13.0	12.8	11.7
Tennessee	8.2	8.0	8.0	6.8	6.6	6.4	13.4	13.0	13.4
Alabama	8.5	8.2	7.9	6.5	6.1	5.9	12.5	12.0	11.8
Mississippi	9.2	8.9	8.7	6.4	6.1	5.8	12.4	12.0	11.9
West South Central:	8.0	7.7	7.2	6.7	6.4	6.0	13.4	13.1	12.7
Arkansas	7.9	7.9	7.6	6.5	6.3	5.9	12.2	12.7	12.6
Louisiana	9.1	8.9	8.5	6.5	6.3	5.8	13.3	12.9	13.0
Oklahoma	7.5	7.2	6.7	6.8	6.6	6.2	14.0	13.2	12.0
Texas	7.8	7.4	6.9	6.7	6.3	6.0	13.7	13.3	12.5
Mountain:	7.7	6.9	6.5	7.5	6.7	6.4	13.8	13.3	11.7
Montana	7.4	6.3	5.6	7.3	6.1	5.5	16.4‡	13.0‡	9.7‡

GEOGRAPHIC DIVISION AND STATE	All Races			White			Black		
	1971–73	1976–78	1981–83[†]	1971–73	1976–78	1981–83[†]	1971–73	1976–78	1981–83[†]
Mountain:	7.7	6.9	6.5	7.5	6.7	6.4	13.8	13.3	11.7
Idaho	6.5	5.6	5.3	6.4	5.6	5.3	4.2[‡]	8.5[‡]	8.5[‡]
Wyoming	8.9	8.3	6.9	8.9	8.1	6.9	18.1[‡]	17.3[‡]	14.2[‡]
Colorado	9.3	8.4	7.9	9.0	8.1	7.6	15.1	14.7	12.7
New Mexico	9.0	8.4	7.6	9.0	8.4	7.6	14.5[‡]	13.6[‡]	11.8[‡]
Arizona	6.7	6.2	6.0	6.5	6.0	5.8	11.1	11.8	11.1
Utah	6.0	5.5	5.5	5.9	5.5	5.4	12.6[‡]	10.9[‡]	10.1[‡]
Nevada	8.6	7.5	6.8	7.6	6.7	6.3	15.7[‡]	13.7[‡]	11.4[‡]
Pacific:	6.5	6.1	5.8	5.9	5.4	5.1	12.2	11.5	11.0
Washington	6.2	5.5	5.2	5.9	5.2	4.9	11.3	9.8	9.9
Oregon	5.8	5.3	4.9	5.6	5.1	4.7	13.6[‡]	11.5[‡]	10.2[‡]
California	6.6	6.2	5.9	5.9	5.5	5.2	12.2	11.6	11.2
Alaska	6.4	5.4	4.8	5.8	5.0	4.4	11.5[‡]	8.9[‡]	7.2[‡]
Hawaii	7.8	7.4	7.1	6.2	6.0	6.0	8.1[‡]	8.9[‡]	9.8[‡]

*Per 100 total live births
[†]For 1979 and later, data are for infants weighing less than 2500 g at birth
[‡]States with fewer than 5,000 live births for the 3-year period
Source: National Center for Health Statistics: Data computed by the Division of Analysis from data compiled by the Division of Vital Statistics

and those of white infants at full-term delivery are greater than they are at premature delivery. During early development, black fetuses are heavier than white ones. But as gestation continues the relationship is reversed: white fetuses become heavier than black (Fig. 3–1). This latter difference may reflect the greater impact of environmental factors (nutrition, maternal smoking and drinking among others) on late fetal development.

The most recent year in which statistical studies were done on a cohort with linked birth and death records is 1960. Fig. 3–2 shows the relationship between birth weight and mortality among white and non-white infants in this group. At low birth weights, white mortality is higher, but the relationship is dramatically reversed at higher birth weights.

The causes of lower or higher birth weight can be viewed in terms of the overall health and health practices of the expectant mother, her nutrition, personal hygiene and her smoking and alcohol consumption. Data from the Surgeon General substantiates that smoking during pregnancy directly retards fetal growth and increases the rates of spontaneous abortion and fetal and neonatal death (Fig. 3–3).

Not surprisingly, other epidemiologic factors associated with birth weight include the number of prenatal visits an expectant mother makes, her education level, maternal age, interval since last birth, whether the birth is a multiple or single one and whether she is married or unmarried. Preventive medicine emphasizes the importance of prenatal care as a way of counteracting the negative

FIG. 3–1.   Percentage of infants of low birth weight by gestation and race: total of 42 reporting states and District of Columbia, 1976

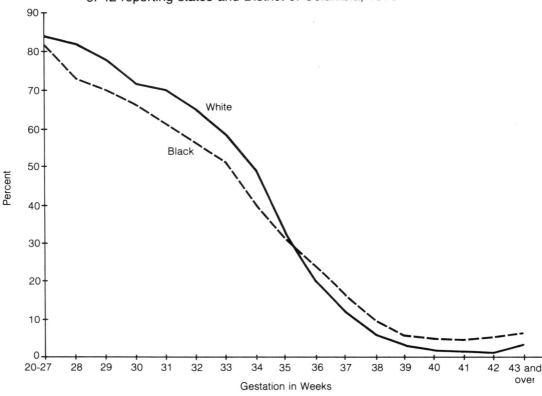

Source: *Vital and Health Statistics*, Series 21, No. 37

impact of several of the factors just cited. Women ignorant of sound health practices and nutrition can be educated during such visits and the complications of pregnancy that develop when the reproductive system is less mature, as in teenage girls, or unreplenished when pregnancies are closely spaced can be medically ameliorated as well.

Prenatal Visits

Various studies show that lack of early prenatal care is associated with low birth weight and infant mortality risk. Both the number of prenatal visits and how soon they are started are directly proportional to fetal and infant health. Ideally, the best birth results are reported for mothers who begin prenatal care during the first trimester and have 13 to 14 prenatal visits. An obvious problem

FIG. 3–2.   Neonatal Mortality by birth weight and race, U.S., 1980

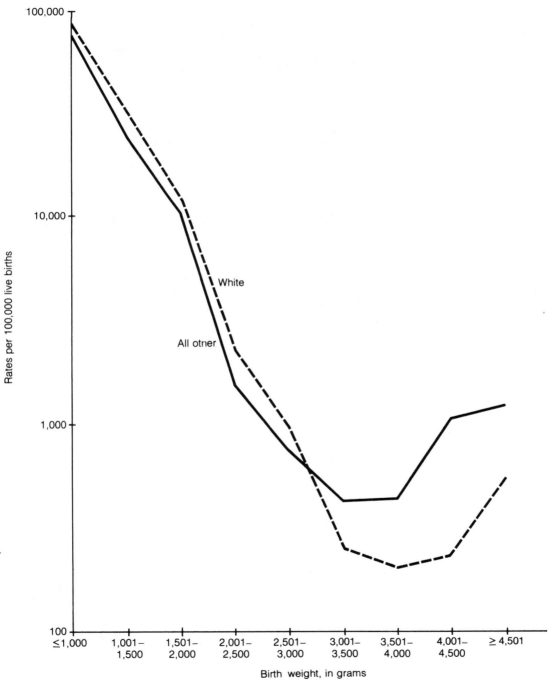

FIG. 3–3.   Risks per 1,000 pregnancies from smoking

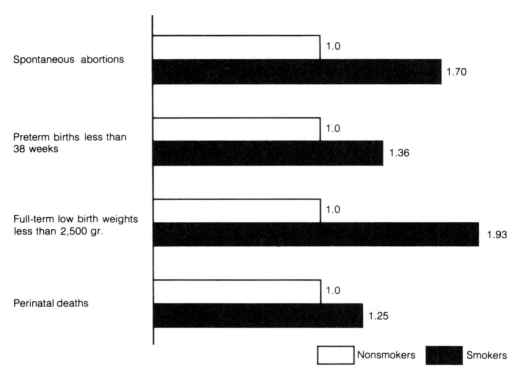

Source: *Report of the Surgeon General, Office on Smoking and Health,* Public Health Service, DHHS

with these correlations is that women who deliver prematurely will by definition have had fewer visits. When premature low birth weight deliveries are eliminated from the data, the importance of prenatal care in infant health is lessened compared to other factors. When the percentage of pregnant women receiving no prenatal care is divided by those starting care in the third trimester for only those infants of 37 weeks' gestation, the percentage ratio of 1.5 (7.9 ÷ 5.1) is lower than the ratio of 2.4 reported for those born at all gestational ages (20.1 ÷ 8.3), including premature babies. In all gestational age groups, the 20.1 percent who had no care was almost 2.5 times the percent that did (Table 3–10).

The prenatal care received seems to vary with such demographic characteristics as educational level, marital status, age, and parity (the number of live births a woman has had). But across all but the first of these variables, black females have received less prenatal care than white. Although the trend for both groups is more care earlier, black females still get less care than white females (Fig. 3–4). Between 1970 and 1979, the proportion of white females

TABLE 3–10. Percentage of Infants of Low Birth Weight, by Time of Initiation of Prenatal Care, Period of Gestation, and Race: Total of 39 reporting States and the District of Columbia, 1975

PERIOD OF GESTATION AND RACE	Care Starting in Third Trimester	No Prenatal Care	Percentage Ratio
All races*			
All gestational ages	8.3	20.1	2.4
37 or more weeks	5.1	7.9	1.5
White:			
All gestational ages	6.9	16.7	2.4
37 or more weeks	4.2	6.2	1.5
Black:			
All gestational ages	12.2	27.4	2.2
37 or more weeks	7.6	11.1	1.5

*Includes races other than white and black
Source: Vital and Health Statistics, Series 21, Vol. 33

receiving early prenatal care rose from 72% to 79%, whereas the porportion of black females rose from 44% to 62%.

The exception to the sizable difference in care received by black and white pregnant females pertains to maternal education. Women with less than 9 years' schooling tend to receive less prenatal care than their more educated counterparts. And this is true for both black and white females. Uneducated females show a narrower racial gap in the prenatal care received than is typical when other factors are considered. In 1975, only 50% of the women with less than 9 years' schooling started care in the first trimester compared with 85.4% of those with 12 years' schooling.

Maternal Education

The incidence of low birth weight infants is about twice as high among unmarried than among married women, even when prenatal care is started during the first trimester. A possible explanation is that, despite medical care, unwed mothers are often less educated than the average expectant mother. As just mentioned, education seems to be critical to infant health. Indeed, governmental data suggest that birth weight outcome depends more on maternal education than on when prenatal care is initiated.

The statistical evidence for low-birth weight babies suggests that education does not merely correlate with prenatal care. It is rather a distinct and more important variable than prenatal care. This observation is supported not only by the fact that more educated women have fewer low birth weight babies than do less educated

FIG. 3–4.   Women beginning prenatal care in the first trimester of pregnancy, according to race: United States. 1970–79.

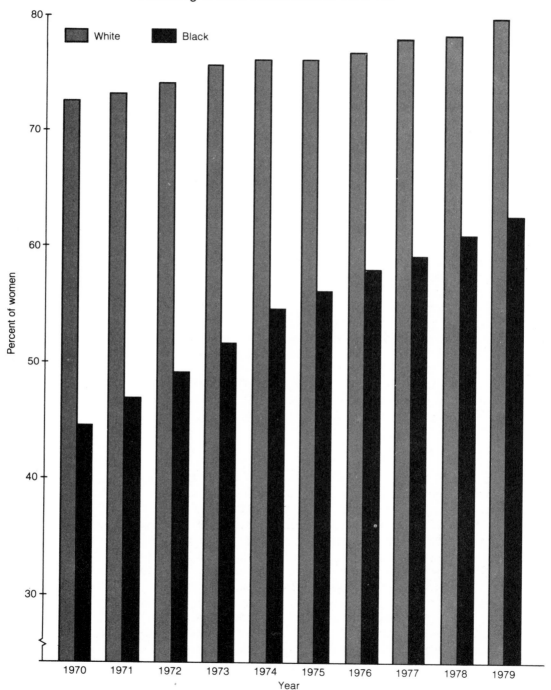

Source: National Center for Health Statistics, Division of Vital Statistics

women receiving the same amount of prenatal care but also that they have fewer low birth weight babies than less educated women receiving *more* prenatal care (Table 3–11).

A certain selection factor may be at work in the data since women in each educational class who delay prenatal care until the seventh month have fewer low-birth weight babies than those starting prenatal care earlier. The possible selection factor is the greater need of women whose pregnancies are problematic to start prenatal care earlier than those having a normal pregnancy. Table 3–12 shows the incidence of low birth weight infants, the level of maternal education, and initiation of prenatal care for pregnant females between 1970 and 1983.

TABLE 3–11.   Percentage of Infants of Low Birth Weight, by Mother's Educational Attainment: Total of 39 Reporting States and the District of Columbia, 1975

MONTH WHEN PRENATAL CARE BEGAN AND CHILD'S RACE		Total	SCHOOLING COMPLETED BY MOTHER				
			0–8	9–11	12	13–15	16 or more
	All races:*	7.5	10.2	10.3	6.9	5.9	5.1
1st and 2nd		6.5	9.1	9.3	6.2	5.5	5.1
3d		6.9	9.5	9.5	6.3	5.6	4.8
4th–6th		8.9	10.3	10.5	8.0	6.8	5.4
7th–9th		8.7	9.6	9.9	7.8	6.6	4.9
No prenatal care		22.6	21.3	24.1	22.0	18.0	15.8
	White:	6.3	8.8	8.5	5.9	5.2	4.7
1st and 2nd		5.7	8.1	7.9	5.6	5.0	4.7
3d		5.9	8.4	8.1	5.5	4.9	4.4
4th–6th		7.2	8.8	8.7	6.6	5.7	4.7
7th–9th		7.3	8.3	8.4	6.5	5.3	3.8
No prenatal care		19.4	19.1	20.8	18.8	14.7	13.7
	Black:	13.2	15.0	14.8	12.1	11.0	9.5
1st and 2nd		12.1	14.0	14.3	11.3	10.6	9.3
3d		12.4	13.9	13.8	11.6	10.6	9.5
4th–6th		13.2	14.8	14.2	12.2	11.1	9.8
7th–9th		12.0	13.9	13.0	10.8	9.8	7.4
No prenatal care		27.7	27.7	28.3	26.8	23.7	22.3

*Includes races other than white and black
Source: *Vital and Health Statistics*, Series 21, No. 33

Presumably, those who are more educated practice better health habits or follow medical advice more closely when receiving prenatal care. Teenage and unwed mothers who have a higher incidence of low birth weight babies are less educated than the average pregnant woman; often simply because they are younger than other expectant mothers.

TABLE 3–12.   Live Births: United States, Selected Years 1970–83 (Data are based on the National Vital Statistics System)

CHILD'S RACE AND SELECTED CHARACTERISTIC	LIVE BIRTHS (%)									
	1970	1975	1976	1977	1978	1979	1980	1981	1982	1983
All races:										
Birth weight*:										
≤ 2500 grams	7.94	7.39	7.26	7.07	7.11	6.94	6.84	6.81	6.75	6.82
≤ 1500 g	1.17	1.16	1.15	1.13	1.17	1.15	1.15	1.16	1.18	1.19
Mother's education:										
< 12 years	30.8	28.6	27.4	26.2	26.1	24.4	23.7	22.9	22.3	21.7
≥ 16 years	8.6	11.4	12.1	12.6	13.1	13.7	14.0	14.8	15.3	15.9
Prenatal care began:										
1st trimester	68.0	72.4	73.5	74.1	74.9	75.9	76.3	76.3	76.1	76.2
3rd trimester or no prenatal care	7.9	6.0	5.7	5.6	5.4	5.1	5.1	5.2	5.5	5.6
Unmarried women	10.7	14.3	14.8	15.5	16.3	17.1	18.4	18.9	19.4	20.3
White:										
Birth weight*:										
≤ 2500 g	6.84	6.26	6.13	5.93	5.94	5.80	5.70	5.67	5.63	5.67
≤ 1500 g	0.95	0.92	0.91	0.89	0.91	0.90	0.90	0.90	0.92	0.93
Mother's education:										
< 12 years	27.0	25.0	23.9	22.9	23.4	21.3	20.7	19.9	19.3	18.7
≥ 16 years	9.5	12.7	13.5	14.0	14.4	15.2	15.6	16.4	17.0	17.7
Prenatal care began:										
1st trimester	72.4	75.9	76.8	77.3	78.2	79.1	79.3	79.4	79.3	79.4
3rd trimester or no prenatal care	6.2	5.0	4.8	4.7	4.5	4.3	4.3	4.3	4.5	4.6
Unmarried women	5.7	7.3	7.7	8.2	8.7	9.4	11.0	11.6	12.1	12.8
Black:										
Birth weight*:										
≤ 2500 g	13.86	13.09	12.97	12.79	12.85	12.55	12.49	12.53	12.40	12.59
≤ 1500 g	2.40	2.37	2.40	2.38	2.43	2.37	2.44	2.47	2.51	2.55
Mother's education:										
< 12 years	51.0	45.1	43.3	41.0	38.5	37.7	36.2	35.4	34.8	34.2
≥ 16 years	2.8	4.4	4.8	5.2	5.7	5.9	6.3	6.6	6.8	6.8
Prenatal care began:										
1st trimester	44.4	55.8	57.7	59.0	60.2	61.6	62.7	62.4	61.5	61.5
3rd trimester or no prenatal care	16.6	10.5	9.9	9.6	9.3	8.9	8.8	9.1	9.6	9.7
Unmarried women	37.6	48.8	50.3	51.7	53.2	54.7	55.3	56.0	56.7	58.2

*Because some of the birth-weight figures are less than 1%, all figures for this category were carried to 2 decimal places. For 1979 and later, data are for infants weighing < 2500 g at birth.
Note: Percents are based only on records for which characteristic is stated.
Source: National Center for Health Statistics: *Vital Statistics of the United States*, Vol. 1, Natality, for data years 1970–80. Public Health Service. Washington. U.S. Government Printing Office; for 1981–83, Public Health Service.

Increased infant risk for very young, uneducated mothers also reflects biologic inadequacy, since their reproductive systems may be incompletely developed. Reproductive inadequacy often affects births following a previous delivery by less than 2 to 4 years. Closely spaced pregnancies and multiple deliveries, e.g., twins and triplets, which occur more often among blacks, may receive less nourishment from a uterus unable to meet excessive reproductive demands.

This biologic factor operates across educational attainment lines. But it is hard to separate it from the low education factor, since teenage, biologically immature mothers, and young mothers who tend to space children more closely than older ones are not only biologically disadvantaged but also typically less educated. Thus, the factor of educational attainment is somewhat confounded by other risk factors such as maternal age and the spacing between pregnancies. In older females, however, it operates independently of biologic factors.

For the several reasons already cited, maternal education more than any other variable, is linked with infant mortality. It is sometimes thought that this variable is just a general socioeconomic variable reflecting whether or not a women can afford prenatal care. However, early studies in England show that even when families earn a good income, i.e., one that would put them in the middle or high middle class, infant mortality can still be high if the mothers are uneducated. Socioeconomic class defined in terms of money is not only a distinct variable from educational level but often inversely related to educational level. Such was the case in the 1950s among English coal miners who were earning higher salaries than the general population. They still had a higher infant mortality than sectors making less.[c]

Maternal awareness of hygiene; safety measures; child care; and the need for proper diet, rest, and medical attention appear to be a key to infant survival beyond merely having the financial ability to secure nutritious food and proper medical care. A belief that having a baby is a natural phenomenon requiring no special modification of health habits, medical advice, or assistance is more common among the less educated. Hence, despite low-cost or affordable care, uneducated women may fail to secure prenatal care or to follow medical advice.

Fertility

Complications of pregnancy, childbirth, and low birth weight occur more often in women who have had three or more children. The lowest risk birth is the second since first births also have a high mortality risk. This is partly due to the trial-and-error that

[c]Norris JN: Health and social class. *Lancet*: 303–305, Feb. 1959

affects first births. Until recently, women have lacked genetic risk information that might have deterred them from becoming pregnant with their first child. When a first-born either was malformed or had genetic defects, women often refrained from further childbearing efforts. This explanation for the higher incidence of birth problems in first over second children was probably truer formerly than it is today when genetic counseling, fetal screening, and abortion are possible before the birth of a first child.

The higher risk of higher order births may seem to relate more to increasing maternal age than to birth order. But this possible explanation is not born out in fact. Risk is greater for each birth higher than two for younger as well as for older women. High order birth risk is, therefore, independent of the risk entailed by advancing maternal age.

Given the high, birth-order risk factor for infant mortality, a declining fertility rate, i.e., the number of live births per 1,000 women age 15 to 44 years, accomplished through reduced family size and fewer high-order births, should be expected to contribute to a decline in infant mortality. The U.S. fertility rate declined markedly from a peak in 1957 to a low in 1976 (Fig. 3–5). The "fertility rate" is not to be confused with "birth rate," which is the number of live births per 100,000 general population, nor with the term "fertility" itself in the sense of the ability to have children.

The total fertility rate dropped by 18.1% between 1960 and 1965 (Table 3–13). But this significant drop was due mostly to a decline in the infants with a birth order higher than one. The number of second-order births declined by 19.9%, the third by 27.2% the fourth by 27.9%, and the fifth or higher by 20.7%.

These declines in higher-order births between 1960 and 1965 coincide with a decline in infant mortality from 1957 that began after steady to slightly rising mortality rates during the high fertility 1950 baby boom years (see Fig. 3–5). Birth order is just one of the factors affecting the mortality rate, but the data support its importance as a contributory factor to reduced infant mortality.

Maternal Age

Another infant mortality risk factor affected by changing fertility and childbearing practices is maternal age. Women younger than age 20 years and older than 35 years are more likely to give birth to low-birth weight, high-risk babies. In recent years, American white females have been deferring marriage and childbearing until they're older.

The live births per 1,000 women age 15 to 19 years dropped dramatically between 1960 and 1975 as it did for all other age

FIG. 3–5. Fertility rates, United States from 1930 to 1983.

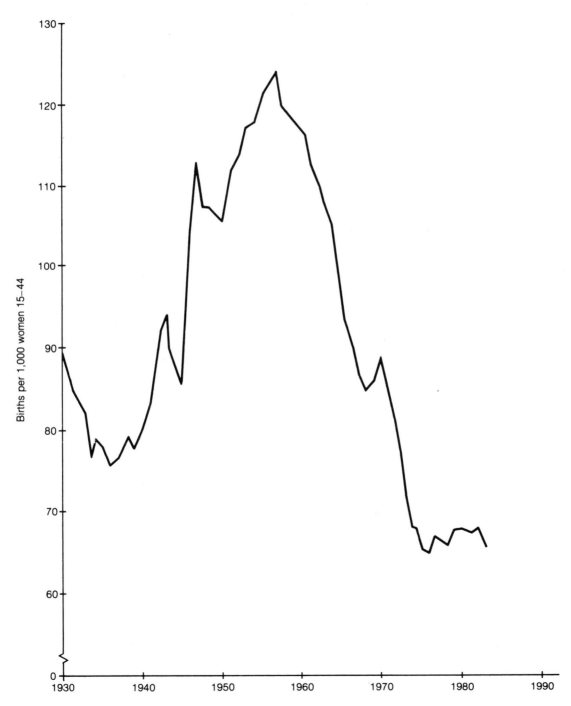

TABLE 3–13.   Birth Rates for Women Age 15–44 Years, According to Live-birth Order and Race: United States, Selected Years 1950–80 (Data are based on the National Vital Statistics System)

RACE AND YEAR	LIVE-BIRTH ORDER*					
	Total	1	2	3	4	5 or more
Total†:						
1950	106.2	33.3	32.1	18.4	9.2	13.2
1955	118.3	32.8	31.8	23.1	13.3	17.3
1960	118.0	31.1	29.2	22.8	14.6	20.3
1965	96.6	29.8	23.4	16.6	10.7	16.1
1970	87.9	34.2	24.2	13.6	7.2	8.7
1975	66.0	28.1	20.9	9.4	3.9	3.7
1976	65.0	27.5	20.8	9.5	3.8	3.4
1977	66.8	28.2	21.6	10.0	3.8	3.2
1978	65.5	27.8	21.1	9.8	3.8	2.9
1979	67.2	28.6	21.6	10.1	3.8	2.9
1980	68.4	29.5	21.8	10.3	3.9	2.9
White:						
1950	102.3	33.3	32.3	17.9	8.4	10.4
1955	113.7	32.6	32.0	22.9	12.6	13.6
1960	113.2	30.8	29.2	22.7	14.1	16.4
1965	91.4	28.9	23.0	16.2	10.2	13.1
1970	84.1	32.9	23.7	13.3	6.8	7.4
1975	62.5	25.7	20.3	8.8	3.5	3.1
1976	61.5	26.3	20.2	8.9	3.4	2.8
1977	63.2	25.9	20.9	9.4	3.4	2.7
1978	61.7	25.6	20.2	9.2	3.3	2.4
1979	63.4	27.4	20.8	9.4	3.4	2.4
1980	64.7	28.4	21.0	9.5	3.4	2.4
Black:						
1960	153.5	33.6	29.3	24.0	18.6	48.0
1965	133.9	35.7	26.2	19.4	14.6	38.0
1970	115.4	43.3	27.1	16.1	10.0	18.9
1975	87.9	36.9	24.2	12.6	6.3	8.0
1976	85.8	35.2	24.4	12.9	6.2	7.2
1977	88.1	35.6	25.5	13.6	6.4	6.9
1978	86.7	34.6	25.4	13.9	6.5	6.4
1979	88.3	35.3	25.8	14.4	6.6	6.2
1980	88.1	35.2	25.7	14.5	6.7	6.0

*Live births per 1,000 women age 15–44 years
†Includes all other races not shown separately
Note: Data are based on births adjusted for underregistration for 1950 and 1955 and on registered births for all other years. Figures for 1960, 1965, and 1970 are based on a 50% sample of births; for 1975–80, they are based on 100% of births in selected states and on a 50% sample of births in all other states. Beginning in 1970, births to U.S. nonresidents are excluded.
Source: National Center for Health Statistics: *Vital Statistics of the United States, 1980*, Vol. 1. Public Health Service, DHHS, Hyattsville, Md.

brackets except 10 to 14 years (Table 3–14). This latter group has seen a 50% rise over its low 0.8% rate of 1960. If the same increase had occurred at a higher rate for this group, it would have had a significant negative impact on overall infant mortality.

TABLE 3–14. Live Births, Crude Birth Rates, and Birth Rates by Age of Mother, According to Race: United States, Selected Years 1950–80 (Data are based on the National Vital Statistics System)

RACE AND YEAR	Live births	Crude birth rate*	Age (in years)								
			10–14	15–17	18–19	20–24	25–29	30–34	35–39	40–44	45–49
					Live births per 1,000 women						
Total[†]:											
1950	3,632,000	24.1	1.0	40.7	132.7	196.6	166.1	103.7	52.9	15.1	1.2
1955	4,097,000	25.0	0.9	44.5	157.9	241.6	190.2	116.0	58.6	16.1	1.0
1960	4,257,850	23.7	0.8	43.9	166.7	258.1	197.4	112.7	56.2	15.5	0.9
1965	3,760,358	19.4	0.8	36.6	124.5	195.3	161.6	94.4	46.2	12.8	0.8
1970	3,731,386	18.4	1.2	38.8	114.7	167.8	145.1	73.3	31.7	8.1	0.5
1975	3,144,198	14.6	1.3	36.1	85.0	113.0	108.2	52.3	19.5	4.6	0.3
1976	3,167,788	14.6	1.2	34.1	80.5	110.3	106.2	53.6	19.0	4.3	0.2
1977	3,326,632	15.1	1.2	33.9	80.9	112.9	111.0	56.4	19.2	4.2	0.2
1978	3,333,279	15.0	1.2	32.2	79.8	109.9	108.5	57.8	19.0	3.9	0.2
1979	3,494,398	15.6	1.2	32.3	81.3	112.8	111.4	60.3	19.5	3.9	0.2
1980	3,612,258	15.9	1.1	32.5	82.1	115.1	112.9	61.9	19.8	3.9	0.2
White:											
1950	3,108,000	23.0	0.4	31.3	120.5	190.4	165.1	102.6	51.4	14.5	1.0
1955	3,485,000	23.8	0.3	35.4	145.7	235.8	186.6	114.0	56.7	15.4	0.9
1960	3,600,744	22.7	0.4	35.5	154.6	252.8	194.9	109.6	54.0	14.7	0.8
1965	3,123,860	18.3	0.3	27.8	111.9	189.0	158.4	91.6	44.0	12.0	0.7
1970	3,091,264	17.4	0.5	29.2	101.5	163.4	145.9	71.9	30.0	7.5	0.4
1975	2,551,996	13.6	0.6	28.0	74.0	108.2	108.1	51.3	18.2	4.2	0.2
1976	2,567,614	13.6	0.6	26.3	70.2	105.3	105.9	52.6	17.8	3.9	0.2
1977	2,691,070	14.1	0.6	26.1	70.5	107.7	110.9	55.3	18.0	3.8	0.2
1978	2,681,116	14.0	0.6	24.9	69.4	104.1	107.9	56.6	17.7	3.5	0.2
1979	2,808,420	14.5	0.6	24.7	71.0	107.0	110.8	59.0	18.3	3.5	0.2
1980	2,898,732	14.9	0.6	25.2	72.1	109.5	112.4	60.4	18.5	3.4	0.2
Black:											
1960	602,264	31.9	4.3	—	—	295.4	218.6	137.1	73.9	21.9	1.1
1965	581,126	27.7	4.3	99.3	227.6	243.1	180.4	111.3	61.9	18.7	1.4
1970	572,362	25.3	5.2	101.4	204.9	202.7	136.3	79.6	41.9	12.5	1.0
1975	511,581	20.7	5.1	85.6	152.4	142.8	102.2	53.1	25.6	7.5	0.5
1976	514,479	20.5	4.7	80.3	142.5	140.5	101.6	53.6	24.8	6.8	0.5
1977	544,221	21.4	4.7	79.6	142.9	144.4	106.4	57.5	25.4	6.6	0.5
1978	551,540	21.3	4.4	75.0	139.7	143.8	105.4	58.3	24.3	6.1	0.4
1979	577,855	22.0	4.6	75.7	140.4	146.3	108.2	60.7	24.7	6.1	0.4
1980	589,616	22.1	4.3	73.6	138.8	146.3	109.1	62.9	24.5	5.8	0.3

*Live births per 1,000 population.
[†]Includes all other races not shown separately.
Note: Data are based on births adjusted for underregistration for 1950 and 1955 and on registered births for all other years. Figures for 1960, 1965, and 1970 are based on a 50% sample of births; for 1975–80, they are based on 100% of births in selected states and on a 50% sample of births in all other States. Beginning in 1970, births to U.S. nonresidents are excluded.
Source: National Center for Health Statistics: *Vital Statistics of the United States, 1980*, Vol. I. Public Health Service, DHHS, Hyattsville, Md.

Since 1975, the fertility rate has increased slightly over earlier lows. But the rates for women age 15 to 19 years, which declined 40% between 1960 and 1975 has dropped more since 1975. At the same time, the rate for women age 20 to 24 years has risen 1.8%; for women 25 to 29 years old, 4.3%; and for women 30 to 35 years old, 18.4%.

These increases in fertility since 1975 for older women occurred at a time when the rate for higher-order births beyond the first born were stable (Table 3–13). The data suggest that women, particularly white women, are having far fewer children than in 1960, limiting the size of their families to one or two children, and delaying the birth of their first and second child until later ages.

In 1979, more than 115,000 first-order births occurred among women in their 30s. The rate jumped from 7.3 first-order births per 1,000 women age 30 to 34 years in 1970 to 12.1 in 1979. At the same time, first-order birth rates for women age 15 to 19 years and 20 to 24 years were falling. Between 1970 and 1973 the first-born rate for women age 20 to 24 years fell from 78.2 to 56.5 per 1,000. It has remained at this latter figure with only a slight increase since 1975.

The recent pattern of reduced family size with postponement of childbearing can also be expected to affect the spacing between births, another risk factor for low birth weight babies.

Teenage Pregnancy

Two other infant mortality risk factors affected by changes in fertility patterns are teenage maternity and marital status. The risk of infant death is higher if a mother is younger than 20 years old or unwed. In 1957, the teenage fertility rate for 18- to 19-year-olds began to drop and in 1972, it began to drop for 15- to 17-year-olds.

Among all teenagers, married or single, the fertility rate has declined more for those age 15 to 19 years among blacks than among whites. So too, the percentage of live births born to black teenagers age 10 to 17 years per 1,000 total live births has also fallen. The same is not true for white teenagers.

Between 1960 and 1980, there has been a 40 percent drop in the fertility rate of teenagers overall, but the drop in fertility for non-teenage women, particularly white women, is even greater. So, the proportion of live births born to white teenagers is rising. The fertility rates of women age 15 to 19 years since 1920 is shown in Fig. 3–6.

The increased fertility rate for females age 10 to 14 years, most of whom are unmarried, has also contributed to a rising rate of babies born out of wedlock. Among older teenagers, age 15 to 19 years, the fertility rate has dropped. But the illegitimacy rate has risen sharply because the marriage rate for women younger than

FIG. 3–6.   Fertility rates of women age 15–19 years, 1920–74.

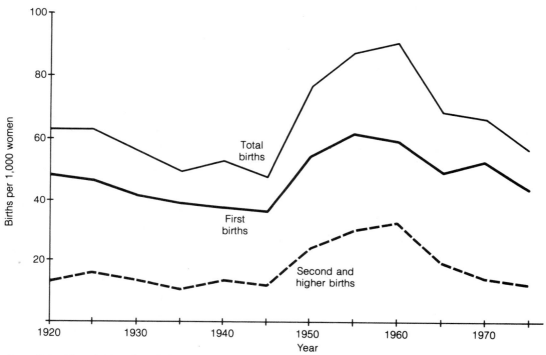

Source: National Center for Health Statistics: Fertility tables for birth cohorts by color, United States 1971–73, DHEW
     PUBLICATION NO (HRA) 76-1152, U. S. Government Printing Office, Washington D.C. 1976, table 34; 1974 data
     supplied by Robert L. Heuser, Chief Natality Statistics Branch, National Center for Health Statistics.

20 has dropped dramatically, much more than the fertility rate decline among these young women.

The marriage rate for women younger than age 20 years has declined from 48% in 1960 to 38% in 1976, according to the census. Data gathered in the National Survey of Family Growth conducted in 1976 by the National Center for Health Statistics reveals that while the fertility rate for unwed women age 15 to 44 years rose 14% between 1960 and 1976, the rate for teenagers increased 57%.

Between 1972 and 1976, of the 6.7 million women under age 25 who were marrying for the first time, 9% had already had one child; and 14% were at least 6 weeks pregnant on their wedding day.

The survey found that about 43% of black teenage wives and 5% of white teenage wives had had a premarital birth. Also, while black teenage single women were more likely than white ones to become pregnant, they were less likely to marry before delivery. This decision to postpone marriage until after the outcome of birth may reflect the higher infant mortality rate for black babies that has existed historically. It also partly accounts for the higher illegitimacy rates among blacks. Although the proportion of unwed births is much higher for blacks than for whites, the increased rate of these births over the 12 years noted has occurred mostly among white teenagers (Table 3–15). Early marriage has declined more among white than among black women.

Although high, the percentage of unmarried black teenagers having a baby among all unmarried black women has been holding fairly steady since 1968. The rate among white teenagers, however, although lower has, as just mentioned, risen sharply. So, too, the percentage of illegitimate births among all births has almost doubled for white teenagers; it has not doubled for black teenagers. The higher base number for blacks, which has still increased more in absolute terms than the white, would be less likely to double. Figure 3–7 shows the trends in illegitimate childbearing for women of diverse ages. The first five line drawings from the bottom show the illegitimate births per 1,000 white women. The top five line drawings, show the number for "all other." The ratio's higher for the latter category except for females age 35 to 44 years. This shows a steep decline for non-white women about the year 1970 that appears on the graph at the same level as the lines for white women age 20 to 24 years and 25 to 29 years.

BIRTH TRAUMA AND DISEASE

As surgical delivery replaces difficult forceps delivery for brow, face, and breech presentations, the "large head" injuries and bruises caused by birth trauma are now far less common than in the past. Fetal monitoring also helps physicians detect cord anomalies during labor, minimizing the risk that the baby will experience oxygen denial.

Increased morbidity from brain damage closely correlates with lower birth weight. Premature infants are particularly susceptible to both the rigors of prolonged labor and perinatal stress with possible oxygen deprivation and the risk of primary post delivery intracerebral hemorrhages for hours or days.

Specific nerve damage leading to various forms of cerebral palsy is associated with oxygen deprivation without hemorrhage. Brain damage from lack of oxygen prevents cerebral-palsy patients from controlling muscle movement. Symptoms can be mild or severe, involving involuntary or erratic, awkward movement; gutteral speech; and grimacing. Generally, intelligence is not impaired;

TABLE 3–15. Selected Measures of Teenage Fertility, According to Age and Race: United States, 1968–79 (Data are based on the National Vital Registration System)

RACE AND YEAR	Age (in years)									
	10–14	15–17	18–19	10–14	15–17	18–19	15–17	18–19	15–17	18–19
	Live births per 1,000 women			Percentage of all live births			Live births to unmarried women[†]		Live births to unmarried women[†]	
Total*:										
1968	1.0	35.1	113.5	0.3	5.5	11.4	14.7	30.0	403.7	201.3
1969	1.0	35.7	112.4	0.3	5.6	11.2	15.2	31.5	412.8	210.7
1970	1.2	38.8	114.7	0.3	6.0	11.3	17.1	32.9	429.8	223.9
1971	1.1	38.3	105.6	0.3	6.4	11.3	17.6	31.7	445.4	232.0
1972	1.2	39.2	97.3	0.4	7.3	11.7	18.6	31.0	458.5	246.8
1973	1.3	38.9	91.8	0.4	7.6	11.7	18.9	30.6	466.9	255.7
1974	1.2	37.7	89.3	0.4	7.4	11.4	19.0	31.4	482.5	270.4
1975	1.3	36.6	85.7	0.4	7.2	11.3	19.5	32.8	513.9	298.1
1976	1.2	34.6	81.3	0.4	6.8	10.8	19.3	32.5	540.2	316.1
1977	1.2	34.5	81.9	0.3	6.4	10.4	20.1	35.0	565.5	343.7
1978	1.2	32.9	81.0	0.3	6.1	10.2	19.5	35.7	574.9	361.6
1979	1.2	33.1	82.6	0.3	5.7	10.0	20.4	37.8	599.6	380.7
White:										
1968	0.4	25.6	100.5	0.1	4.2	10.5	6.2	16.8	234.4	127.4
1969	0.4	26.4	99.2	0.1	4.3	10.2	6.6	17.0	240.3	129.0
1970	0.5	29.2	101.5	0.1	4.6	10.4	7.5	17.6	252.0	135.0
1971	0.5	28.6	92.4	0.1	4.9	10.4	7.4	15.9	251.7	131.7
1972	0.5	29.4	84.5	0.2	5.7	10.7	8.7	15.1	264.4	136.7
1973	0.6	29.5	79.6	0.2	6.0	10.6	8.5	15.0	276.4	142.6
1974	0.6	29.0	77.7	0.2	5.9	10.4	8.9	15.4	294.2	150.1
1975	0.6	28.3	74.4	0.2	5.8	10.3	9.7	16.6	329.6	171.9
1976	0.6	26.7	70.7	0.2	5.4	9.9	9.9	17.0	357.4	187.9
1977	0.6	26.5	71.1	0.2	5.1	9.4	10.7	18.8	389.2	209.5
1978	0.6	25.4	70.1	0.2	4.9	9.3	10.5	19.5	400.9	224.4
1979	0.6	25.3	71.8	0.2	4.6	9.1	11.1	21.2	424.3	242.7
Black:										
1968	4.7	98.2	206.1	1.2	13.1	16.6	—	—	—	—
1969	4.8	96.9	202.5	1.2	13.1	16.7	72.3	129.1	720.9	482.9
1970	5.2	101.4	204.9	1.3	13.4	16.6	77.9	136.4	759.6	521.4
1971	5.1	99.7	193.8	1.3	14.0	16.4	80.9	136.3	796.3	560.3
1972	5.1	99.9	181.7	1.4	15.5	17.0	82.9	129.8	810.1	590.2
1973	5.4	96.8	169.5	1.5	15.8	17.1	81.9	123.0	825.6	603.8
1974	5.0	91.0	162.0	1.4	15.4	17.1	79.4	124.9	848.0	638.3
1975	5.1	86.6	156.0	1.4	14.6	16.8	77.7	126.8	874.0	676.0
1976	4.7	81.5	146.8	1.3	13.9	16.0	74.6	121.6	897.4	709.0
1977	4.7	81.2	147.6	1.2	13.1	15.4	74.3	125.9	904.7	746.4
1978	4.4	76.6	145.0	1.1	12.2	15.2	70.3	124.3	909.1	764.8
1979	4.6	77.3	146.7	1.1	11.7	14.7	72.5	128.8	928.7	788.7

*Includes all other races not shown separately
[†]Per 1,000 unwed mothers
[‡]Per 1,000 total live births
Note: Data are based on births adjusted for underregistration for 1950 and 1955 and on registered births for all other years. Figures for 1960, 1965, and 1970 are based on a 50% sample of births; for 1975–79, they are based on 100% of births in selected states and on a 50% sample of births in all other states. Beginning in 1970, births to U.S. nonresidents are excluded.
Source: Division of Vital Statistics, National Center for Health Statistics: Selected data.

FIG. 3–7.   Estimated birth rates for unmarried women by age of mother and color: United States, 1940, 1950 and 1955–76

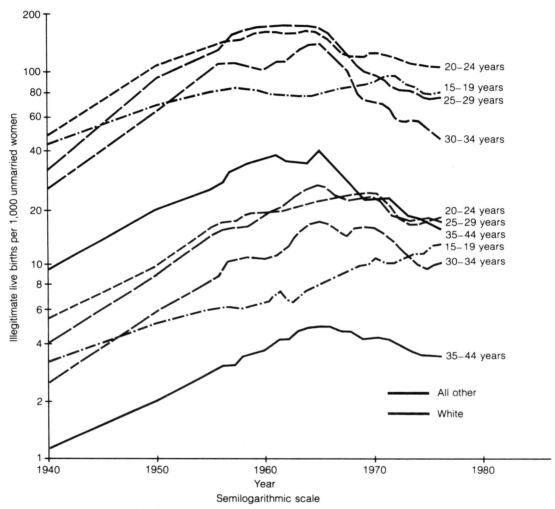

Source: *Vital and Health Statistics*, Series 21, No. 36

with or without therapy many patients lead productive lives. Cerebral-palsy studies show an association between marked prematurity, abnormal presentation, and perinatal asphyxia.

The United Cerebral Palsy Association estimates that 3.5 cases of cerebral palsy occur per 1,000 live births—15,000 babies annually. The estimate is lower than estimates given 25 to 30 years ago of between 2 to 6 per 1,000 live births. The Association believes that cases are decreasing because of modern pregnancy management and delivery of women with an Rh-negative factor, a cause of athetoid cerebral palsy (see Glossary). Spastic diplegia, paralysis on both sides of the body, and the other types of cerebral palsy seen in low birth weight babies and babies injured during birth is falling due to perinatal units and the advances in managing high-risk infants.

Despite the prevention of birth trauma through increased use of cesarean delivery, other conditions such as maternal bleeding or intrauterine growth retardation associated with toxemia are not preventable through cesarean section. Toxemia is typically associated with preexisting cardiovascular or renal disease. It's characterized by hypertension, fluid retention in the tissues, and convulsions or coma in its severest form and is responsible for brain damage. A cesarean section can attenuate a toxemia that is becoming progressively severe, thereby protecting the mother's life. But the baby, if premature, may still not survive.

On the other hand, a cesarean delivery even when efficacious, poses its own hazards to the baby if gestational age is not correctly assessed. Fetal lung immaturity can lead to respiratory distress syndrome (RDS). Indeed, at all gestational ages, cesarean delivery is associated with a higher RDS incidence.

Respiratory distress syndrome is the equivalent of the disorder called hyaline membrane disease. It occurs mainly in babies of less than 36 weeks' gestation; its signs and symptoms include rapid breathing, grunting, and cyanosis. Records of all births in Norway between 1967 and 1973 indicated an RDS incidence after uncomplicated cesarean delivery of 7.9 per 1,000 compared to 1.7 per 1,000 in uncomplicated vaginal delivery.[d] This equals a relative risk of 4.6 ($p < 0.05$). A relative risk measure as used here is the incidence in the cesarean group divided by or relative to the incidence in the vaginal delivery group.

Also occurring more often in children born to diabetic mothers, RDS is the most common cause of neonatal mortality. It's responsible for 4,000 infant deaths annually. Treatment consists of thorough respiratory support, maintaining fluid and electrolyte balances, and nutritional assistance.

POSTNEONATAL CAUSES OF DISEASE

By 1982, two-thirds of all infant deaths in developed countries occurred in the first week of life. They were due to congenital

[d]U.S. Dept. of Health and Human Services, NIH pub. No. 82-2067 "Cesarean Childbirth," p. 321

anomalies, birth trauma, or other perinatal conditions. Although dramatic gains were made in reducing infant neonatal mortality during the 1970's, most of the strides made in this century by developed countries have been in reducing postneonatal mortality through greatly improving environmental conditions. Such improvements include stabilizing food supplies, purifying water supplies, effectively disposing of sewage, pasteurizing milk, and administering vaccines and antibiotics.

SUDDEN INFANT DEATH SYNDROME

At present, one of the leading causes of postneonatal mortality in the United States is sudden infant death syndrome (SIDS). It's suspected when a seemingly healthy infant dies suddenly and unexpectedly, and no other cause of death can be determined on autopsy examination. An estimated 5,000 to 7,000 cases occur yearly. The Department of Health and Human Services has awarded several grants to permit the gathering of more accurate data about SIDS.

INFECTIONS

Gains in postneonatal survival in developed countries, such as Canada, the United States, Japan, Australia, New Zealand, and those of continental Europe, have not occurred to the same extent in undeveloped countries. Since 1965, public health and medical programs initiated in undeveloped countries have helped to lower overall infant mortality rates—sometimes at a rate exceeding the decline experienced by developed countries earlier in this century. Nevertheless, infant mortality although often based on rough estimates, still seems to be much higher than in developed countries because of various geographic, political, cultural and socioeconomic conditions. The political situation of starving Ethiopians is an extreme and prime example.

The causes of death in less developed countries are chiefly postneonatal—pneumonia, influenza, diarrhea, and malnutrition—rather than neonatal causes, such as congenital anomalies. Efforts to disseminate information on oral rehydration have been made to minimize deaths from diarrhea. The United States has also initiated programs and education for women in third-world countries in the correct use of prepared infant formulas, which often replace breast feeding. The mortality rate for infants up to age 1 year in several underdeveloped countries is shown in Table 3–16.

TABLE 3–16.   Infant Mortality in Underdeveloped Countries, 1975–1980: Average Estimates

Country	Death Rate per 1,000 Live Births
Boliva	138.2
China	48.7
Haiti	120.0
Indonesia	125.0
Jordan	75.1
Liberia	159.2
Madagascar	102.0
Phillipines	58.9
Saudi Arabia	126.1
South Africa	100.6
Yemen	169.6

Source: U.N. Demographic Yearbook, 1982

ACCIDENTS

Some analysts assert that death estimates for underdeveloped countries show influenza/pneumonia to be the leading causes of childhood death followed by gastritis, enteritis, and accidents. In developed countries, the leading cause of childhood death is accident followed by influenza/pneumonia and congenital anomalies.

Between 1950 and 1979, the death rate for American children age 1 to 5 years for nonmotor-vehicle accidents fell by 32%. The rate for motor-vehicle accidents remained stable. Since there was a 53% drop in the death rate for this age group overall, due largely to reduction of disease, the proportion of accidental deaths today is 15% higher than in 1950.

In 1979, the death rate for nonmotor-vehicle accidents, e.g., fire and drowning, was 1.6 times greater for boys than for girls and 1.9 times greater for black children than white. Even the motor-vehicle death rate was 15% higher for boys than for girls and 17% higher for blacks than for whites.

Yet, there has been a greater *absolute* reduction in the death rate of black children than of white since 1950, particularly from pneumonia and influenza, congenital anomalies, and cancers such as leukemia. Still, by 1979 the death rate for white children was one-half as high as it was for black children. The overall change in death rates for these several causes including accidents is shown in Fig. 3–8.

FIG. 3–8. Death rates for children 1–4 years of age, according to leading causes of death, United States, 1950–1979

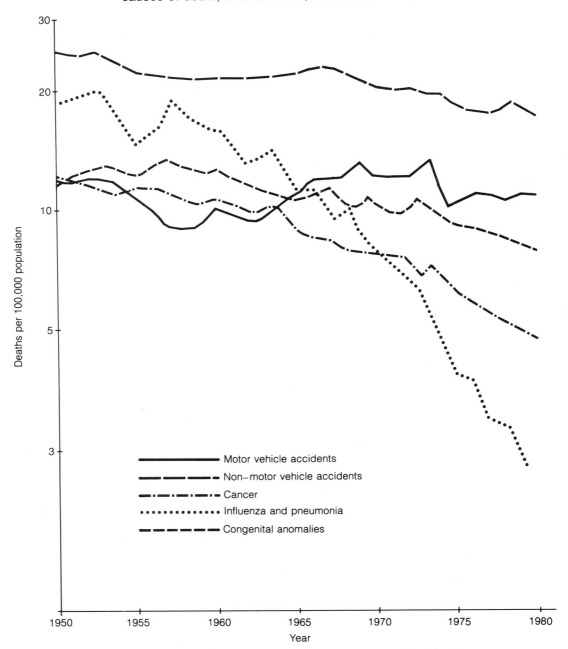

Causes of death are assigned according to the International List of Causes of Death. Because of the decennial revisions and changes in rules for cause-of-death selection there may be some lack of comparability from one revision to the next. The beginning dates of the revisions are 1949, 1958, 1968 and 1979.

Source: National Center for Health Statistics, Division of vital Statistics

LEAD POISONING

Another major contributor to illness in American children age 6 months to 5 years is lead poisoning. The Centers for Disease Control reported that in the first 6 months of fiscal 1981, about 20,000 children were being treated for lead poisoning. They suffered from impaired hematopoiesis (blood cell production) and neuropsychologic deficits.

The main avenue of exposure and absorption in children, particularly those living in old urban housing who are mostly black seems to be ingestion. They also absorb higher levels per body weight through inhalation than do adults. Encouragingly, results of a government survey of samples taken between 1976 and 1980 show marked decreases in average serum lead levels, from 15.8 mcg/dl to 10.0 mcg/dl. This 37% fall for all respondents was not associated with changes in geographic location or laboratory error. But it does correspond to government regulation of car emissions.

Because of the concern about this public-health problem, the NHANES II proposed to determine population serum lead levels based on samples drawn from 16,563 persons, including children. Differences among black and white children by age and sex are shown in Fig. 3–9. The statistically significant differences are racial, with black children having higher serum lead levels than white ones. Urban children and those from lower-income households also had higher lead levels.

The NHANES II data indicate an estimated 4% of all American children 6 months to 5 years have elevated serum lead levels. Not surprisingly, 12.2% of all black children have levels higher than the CDC guideline of 30 mcg/dl; only 2% of white children do. Information available only recently on Spanish-American children show that only 1% have serum lead contamination. This is lower than the rate for white children. Data for the Spanish-American group has been available since 1980 after air pollution regulation reduced lead levels for the population as a whole. Much attention has been focused on the ingestion of lead-based paint, common in older houses as a cause of the higher lead levels in black children detected in the 1970s. But the current low rate in Spanish-American children who often live in similar housing suggests that the high black rates may have been due more to vehicle exhaust fumes than to paint ingestion.

Research also links vehicle exhaust fumes to a greater susceptibility to respiratory infections in children and adults.

FIG. 3–9.   Serum lead levels by (A) sex and (B) race.

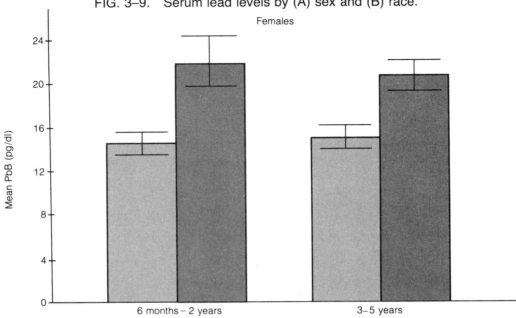

Source: National Health and Nutrition Examination Survey, National Center for Health Statistics.

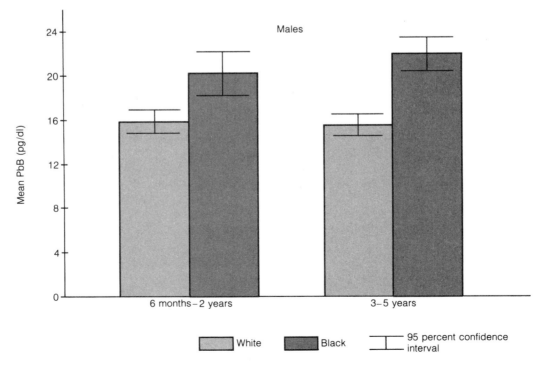

Mean blood levels: (Pb5) of children ages 6 months–
five years, United States, 1976–80

Source: *Vital and Health Statistics Advancedata*, No. 79, May 1982

Obstetrics   4

The U.S. maternal mortality rate per 100,000 has fallen sharply since 1950, from 84 deaths to 8 in 1980 (Fig. 1–1). The Department of Health and Human Services has set a goal of no more than 5 deaths per 100,000 by 1990.

The maternal mortality rate for all other women is still about four times higher than that of white women in the United States as of 1978 (Table 4–1). In 1915 to 1919, the disparity was less between them although both had much higher rates, with 700.3 for white women and 1253.5 for all others.

The geographical differences in maternal mortality for white and non-white women for 1976 to 1978 are shown in Table 4–2.

MATERNAL DISEASE AND DEATH

Death rates for women in several countries and the United States between 1978 and 1980 are shown in Table 4–3. The relatively complete data for 1978 reveal that recent rates for developed countries like Denmark, Switzerland, and the United States are low. However, a few, such as Luxembourg and Romania at 73.7 and 129.2 per 100,000, have rates nearly as high as or higher than the less developed countries of Mexico at 103.4 and Guatemala at 120.8 per 100,000.

73

FIG. 4–1. Maternal mortality rates: 1950–81.

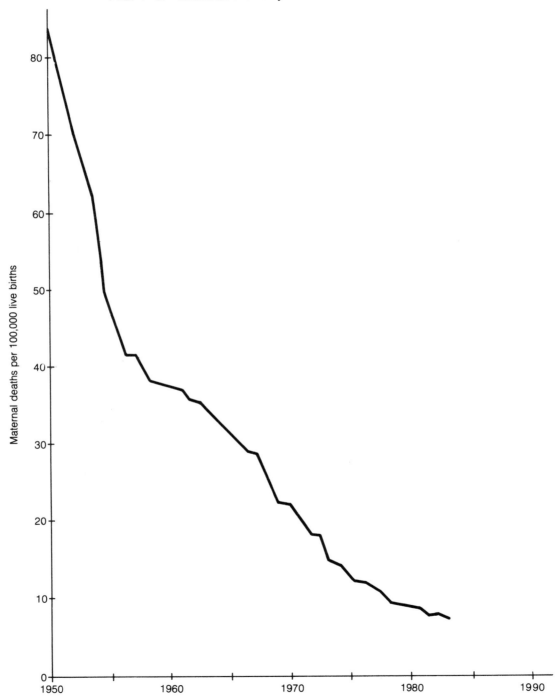

TABLE 4–1. Maternal Mortality Rates by Color: Birth-Registration States or United States, 1915–78 (Prior to 1933, data are for birth-registration States only. Rates per 100,000 live births in specified group. Deaths are classified according to the International Classification of Diseases in use at the time)

YEAR	TOTAL¶	WHITE	ALL OTHER	YEAR	TOTAL¶	WHITE	ALL OTHER
1978★	9.6	6.4	23.0	1955	47.0	32.8	130.3
1977★	11.2	7.7	26.0	1954	52.4	37.2	143.8
1976★	12.3	9.0	26.5	1953	61.1	44.1	166.1
1975★	12.8	9.1	29.0	1952	67.8	43.9	188.1
1974★	14.6	10.0	35.1	1951	75.0	54.9	201.3
1973★	15.2	10.7	34.6	1950	83.3	61.1	221.6
1972★,†	18.8	14.3	38.5				
1971★	18.8	13.0	45.3	1949	90.3	68.1	234.8
1970★	21.5	14.4	55.9	1948	116.5	85.4	301.0
1969	22.2	15.5	55.7	1947	134.5	108.6	334.6
1968	24.5	18.6	63.8	1946	156.7	130.7	358.9
1967	28.0	19.5	69.5	1945	207.2	172.1	454.8
1966	29.1	20.2	72.4				
1965	31.6	21.0	83.7	1944	227.9	189.4	506.0
1964	33.3	22.3	89.9	1943	245.2	210.5	509.9
1963‡	35.8	24.0	96.9	1942	258.7	221.8	544.0
1962‡	35.2	23.8	95.9	1941	316.5	266.0	678.1
1961	36.9	24.9	101.3	1940	376.0	319.8	773.5
1960	37.1	26.0	97.9	1935–39	493.9	439.9	875.5
1959	37.4	25.8	102.1	1930–34★★	636.0	575.4	1,080.7
1958	37.6	28.3	101.8	1925–29	668.6	615.0	1,183.7
1957	41.0	27.5	118.3	1920–24	689.5	649.2	1,134.3
1956	40.9	28.7	110.7	1915–19	727.9	700.3	1,253.5

★Excludes deaths of U.S. nonresidents
†Deaths based on a 50% sample.
‡Figures by color exclude data for residents of New Jersey.
★★For 1932–34, Mexicans are included with "All other".
¶The rates for "white" and "all other" cannot be added mathematically for the "total" rate, since rates are percentages based on different sized populations
Source: *Vital Statistics of the United States*, Vol. II. *Mortality* 1978

TABLE 4–2. Maternal Mortality Rates by Color: United States, Each Division and State, 1976–78 (3-Year Average; Maternal deaths are those assigned to complications of pregnancy, childbirth, and the puerperium, cagetory numbers 630–678 of the Eighth Revision International Classification of Diseases, Adapted, 1965. Rates per 100,000 live births in specified group, 1976–78. Asterisk indicates rate based on a frequency of less than 20)

DIVISION AND STATE	TOTAL	WHITE	ALL OTHER	DIVSION AND STATE	TOTAL	WHITE	ALL OTHER
United States	11.0	7.7	25.1	South Atlantic:			
				Delaware	*23.6	*10.3	*65.9
				Maryland	*7.3	*4.4	*14.0
Geographic divisions:				District of Columbia	*24.0	—	*28.4
New England	6.4	6.3	*8.7	Virginia	10.6	*7.4	*19.8
Middle Atlantic	11.6	7.2	29.9	West Virginia	*9.1	*9.5	—
East North Central	10.3	7.3	25.6	North Carolina	11.7	*7.1	*21.4
West North Central	8.6	7.5	*20.0	South Carolina	16.3	*8.0	*28.4
South Atlantic	13.0	7.2	26.1	Georgia	17.7	*7.6	35.3
East South Central	14.7	7.7	33.0	Florida	12.8	*7.1	27.6
West South Central	13.0	8.9	27.8				

DIVISION AND STATE	TOTAL	WHITE	ALL OTHER	DIVSION AND STATE	TOTAL	WHITE	ALL OTHER
Mountain	9.4	8.0	*23.1				
Pacific	9.3	8.7	12.4				
				East South Central:			
				Kentucky	*9.3	*5.2	*48.8
New England:				Tennessee	14.8	*7.9	*39.0
Maine	*6.4	*6.5	—	Alabama	18.9	*9.4	36.1
New Hampshire	*11.2	*11.4	—	Mississippi	15.8	*10.2	*21.9
Vermont	*23.9	*24.1	—				
Massachusetts	*4.9	*4.8	*6.3	West South Central:			
Rhode Island	*8.8	*9.6	—	Arkansas	*12.4	*9.0	*22.1
Connecticut	*3.7	*2.1	*13.9	Louisiana	17.3	*3.8	37.6
				Oklahoma	*11.8	*8.3	*26.9
Middle Atlantic:				Texas	12.0	10.2	21.4
New York	10.8	6.8	24.6				
New Jersey	12.2	*6.4	34.2	Mountain:			
Pennsylvania	12.5	8.2	39.3	Montana	*7.6	*5.7	*24.1
				Idaho	*5.4	*5.5	—
East North Central:				Wyoming	*32.9	*30.3	*80.1
Ohio	11.5	8.3	31.2	Colorado	*6.2	*4.2	*33.7
Indiana	8.8	*5.9	*32.4	New Mexico	*5.8	*7.0	—
Illinois	9.8	6.5	20.7	Arizona	*9.6	*5.7	*29.8
Michigan	10.0	6.6	*25.9	Utah	*12.5	*12.0	*26.8
Wisconsin	10.9	*9.6	*26.3	Nevada	9.7	*7.7	*20.8
West North Central:							
Minnesota	*6.2	*5.9	*12.0				
Iowa	*7.6	*5.5	*72.5	Pacific:			
Missouri	9.3	*7.2	*20.1	Washington	*5.9	*5.9	*6.0
North Dakota	*9.0	*6.5	*38.4	Oregon	*6.3	*6.7	—
South Dakota	*5.6	*6.4	—	California	10.5	9.5	15.4
Nebraska	*10.8	*10.1	*21.5	Alaska	*7.9	*11.1	—
Kansas	*11.9	*12.2	*9.4	Hawaii	*4.0	—	*5.4

Source: *Vital Statistics of the U.S.*, Vol II *Mortality* 1978

TABLE 4–3.   Maternal Mortality Rate By Most Recent Year for Selected Countries

COUNTRY	RATE PER	YEAR (19)
Barbados	70.2	'79
Bulgaria	21.1	'80
Denmark	8.0	'78
Guatemala	120.8	'78
Kuwait	14.5	'79
Luxembourg	73.7	'78
Mexico	103.4	'78
Romania	129.2	'78
Sweden	6.4	'78
Switzerland	18.2	'78
United States	9.6	'78
Yugoslavia	21.8	'79
Zimbabwe	37.1	'79

Source: *U.N. Demographic Yearbook*, 1984

In 1983, 8 women per 100,000 live births died in the United States from pregnancy complications, childbirth, and the puerperium (confinement after labor). This represents a remarkable gain in years of life for women who, as recently as 1950, were dying in childbirth at a rate of 73.8 per 100,000. The risk of death rises with age and is generally higher for black women than for white (Table 4–4).

TABLE 4–4. Maternal Mortality Rates for Complications of Pregnancy, Childbirth, and the Puerperium, According to Race and Age: United States, Selected Years 1950–83 (Data are based on the National Vital Statistics System)

RACE AND AGE (IN YEARS)	1950★	1960★	1970	1979	1980	1981	1982	1983
All races:	Number of deaths per 100,000 live births							
All ages, age-adjusted	73.8	32.2	21.5	10.2	9.6	8.9	8.0	8.0
All ages, crude	83.3	37.1	21.5	9.6	9.2	8.5	7.9	8.0
Under 20	70.7	22.7	18.9	6.2	7.6	7.6	6.5	5.4
20–24	47.6	20.7	13.0	7.5	5.8	6.5	4.5	7.5
25–29	63.5	29.8	17.0	7.6	7.7	6.6	7.6	6.6
30–34	107.7	50.3	31.6	12.8	13.6	11.4	11.4	9.1
35–39	191.2	92.8	71.0	33.3	31.3	22.6	18.5	20.0
40 and over[†]	335.8	147.0	118.6	82.6	65.9	65.3	61.8	27.0
White:								
All ages, age-adjusted	53.2	22.4	14.5	6.6	7.0	6.5	5.7	5.9
All ages, crude	61.1	26.0	14.4	6.4	6.7	6.3	5.8	5.9
Under 20	44.9	14.8	13.9	3.3	5.9	4.3	4.1	4.4
20–24	35.7	15.3	8.4	4.5	4.3	5.3	3.1	4.9
25–29	45.0	20.3	11.2	5.8	5.5	5.1	5.5	5.2
30–34	75.9	34.3	18.8	8.7	9.4	8.7	9.1	6.0
35–39	144.0	64.1	48.6	23.8	21.2	16.2	13.9	15.6
40 and over[†]	286.4	110.8	97.6	42.8	53.9	42.8	40.2	29.8
Black:								
All ages, age-adjusted	—	92.1	64.2	28.2	24.0	22.1	20.0	19.3
All ages, crude	—	103.6	59.8	25.1	21.5	20.4	18.2	18.3
Under 20	—	54.8	31.8	13.8	12.8	16.8	12.3	7.0
20–24	—	56.9	41.0	22.3	13.4	13.0	11.6	20.2
25–29	—	92.8	63.8	20.0	21.4	17.9	22.3	16.0
30–34	—	150.6	115.6	44.0	41.9	34.2	22.9	31.1
35–39	—	280.2	193.3	88.2	91.7	65.4	51.5	44.7
40 and over[†]	—	369.8	240.7	183.5	119.2	167.2	166.6	25.0

★Includes deaths of U.S. nonresidents
†Rates computed by relating deaths of women 40 years and over to live births to women 40–49 years
Sources: National Center for Health Statistics: *Vital Statistics of the United States*, Vol. II, Mortality, Part A, 1950–83. Public Health Service. Washington. U.S. Government Printing Office; *Vital Statistics of the United States*, Vol. I, Natality, 1950–83. Public Health Service. Washington. U.S. Government Printing Office; Data computed by the Division of Analysis from data compiled by the Division of Vital Statistics; U.S. Bureau of the Census: Population estimates and projections. *Current Population Reports*. Series P-25, No. 499. Washington. U.S. Government Printing Office, May 1973

Delivering women made up 9.9% of all hospital discharges except newborn infants in 1980. About one-half of them developed a complication (Table 4–5). Forceps or vacuum extractor delivery and obstetric trauma were the two most common diagnoses for women with complicated deliveries. Table 4–5 shows the various diagnoses occurring in complicated deliveries, together with the average length of stay for each. Trauma usually involved laceration or other injury to the perineum or vulva. Most of the complications are associated with a stay longer than the average 3.0 days for women with normal, noncomplicated deliveries.

Table 4–6 shows the frequency of various medical interventions undertaken in deliveries whether very complicated or near-normal. Some procedures, such as an episiotomy to prevent tearing as the baby emerges, are routine even when the delivery is not considered complicated.

CESAREAN SECTION

Many pregnancy and delivery complications are indication for a cesarean section. As with any major surgical procedure, a cesarean requires longer hospitalization beyond whatever the initial complication may have required. In 1980, of the total procedures, 15.6% were cesarean sections. This constituted 619,000 operations performed on 16.5% of all mothers and 32.2% of all women with complicated deliveries.

The frequency of cesarean has increased greatly. In 1965, only 5%, or 174,000 deliveries, were by cesarean section. The U.S. cesarean birth rate increased three-fold in the 1970s—from 5.5% (195,000 operations) in 1970 to 15.2% (510,000) in 1978. The trend toward cesarean section as a childbirth procedure affects women of all types in all geographic areas (Table 4–7, Fig. 4–2).

Increasing use of cesarean delivery is a trend in other countries too. In the 1970s, Canada had an increase from 7.5% in 1972 and 1973 to 13.9% in 1979. France, England, Norway, and the Netherlands have also had an increase in cesarean sections, but their rates are lower than those for the United States and Canada (Fig. 4–3).

Cesarean section raises the risk of maternal morbidity and mortality and disadvantages some premature infants. Hence, its increasing use has aroused criticism and scrutiny. The National Institute of Child Health and Human Development convened a task force to investigate the reasons for the marked increase in cesarean delivery. It found several factors that may be contributing

TABLE 4-5. Number and percentage Distribution and Average Length of Stay by First Listed Obstetrical Diagnosis and Number and Percentage Distributor by All-listed Diagnoses for Women Discharged with Complicated Deliveries, United States 1980 (Discharges from short-stay non-Federal hospital Diagnostic groupings and code numbers from the International Classification of Diseases 9th Revision Clinical Modification)

| DIAGNOSIS AND ICD-9-CM CODE | | WOMEN WITH COMPLICATED DELIVERIES: | | | | |
| | | First-listed diagnosis | | | All-listed diagnoses | |
		Number (in thousands)	% distribution	Average stay (in days)	Number (in thousands)	% distribution
All obstetrical diagnoses	640–648, 651–676	1,921	100.0	4.5	2,647	100.0
Forceps or vacuum extractor delivery without mention of indication	669.5	350	18.2	3.3	350	13.2
Obstetrical trauma	664–665	297	15.4	3.1	393	14.8
Trauma to perineum and vulva during delivery	664	241	12.6	3.0	308	11.6
First-degree perineal laceration	664.0	60	3.1	2.9	71	2.7
Second-degree perineal laceration	664.1	50	2.6	2.8	62	2.3
Third-degree perineal laceration	664.2	51	2.7	3.3	68	2.6
Fourth-degree perineal laceration	664.3	46	2.4	3.4	60	2.3
Other and unspecified trauma to perineum and vulva	664.4–664.9	34	1.8	2.7	47	1.8
Laceration of cervix and high vaginal laceration	665.3–665.4	39	2.0	3.1	59	2.2
Other obstetric trauma	665.0–665.2, 665.5–665.9	17	0.9	3.7	26	1.0
Uterine scar from previous surgery	654.2	169	8.8	5.9	192	7.2
Early onset of delivery	644.2	135	7.0	4.8	154	5.8
Fetopelvic disproportion	653.4	113	5.9	5.9	153	5.8
Hypertension complicating pregnancy, childbirth, and the puerperium	642	105	5.5	6.1	151	5.7
Breech presentation	652.1–652.2, 669.6	88	4.6	4.9	120	4.5
Rupture of membranes	658.1–658.3	87	4.5	4.4	130	4.9
Cesarean delivery, without mention of indication	669.7	50	2.6	6.1	50	1.9
Postpartum hemorrhage	666	36	1.6	3.2	54	2.1
Umbilical cord complications	663	35	1.6	3.6	67	2.5
Anemia	648.2	32	1.7	3.9	71	2.7
Fetal distress	656.3	32	1.7	4.8	64	2.4
Antepartum hemorrhage, abruption placentae, and placenta previs	641	28	1.5	6.4	53	2.0
Uterine inertia	661.0–661.2	24	1.3	4.5	50	1.9
Infections of genitourinary tract in pregnancy	646.6	20	1.1	4.7	56	2.1
Other obstetric complications	Residual	320	16.7	4.9	539	20.4

Source: *Vital and Health Statistics Advancedata*, No. 83 Oct. 1982

TABLE 4–6.   Number and Percentage Distrbution of All-listed Procedures for Women Discharged with Deliveries by Type of Procedure: United States 1980 (Discharges from short-stay non-Federal hospitals; Procedure groupings and code numbers from the International Classification of Diseases 9th Revision Clinical Modificiation)

PROCEDURE AND ICD-9-CM CODE		ALL-LISTED PROCEDURES	
		Number (in thousands)	% distribution
All procedures		3,972	100.0
All obstetrical procedures*	72–75	3,526	88.8
Low forceps operation with and without episiotomy	72.0–72.1	482	12.1
Extraction procedures to assist delivery	72.2–72.5, 72.7–72.9, 73.2	127	3.2
Midforceps operation with and without episiotomy	72.2	38	1.0
Forceps rotation of fetal head	72.4	31	0.8
Breech extraction	72.5	21	0.5
Vacuum extraction	72.7	22	0.6
Other extraction procedures to assist delivery	Residual	16	0.4
Episiotomy	72.1, 72.21, 72.31, 72.71, 73.6	2,012	50.7
Episiotomy only	73.6	1,543	38.8
Low forceps operation with episiotomy	72.1	428	10.8
Other instrumental delivery with episiotomy	72.21, 72.31, 72.71	41	1.0
Artificial rupture of membranes	73.0	120	3.0
Other procedures to assist delivery	72.6, 73.1	117	2.9
Cesarean section	74.0–74.2, 74.4–74.9	619	15.6
Diagnostic amniocentesis and fetal monitoring	75.1, 75.34	119	3.0
Manual removal of retained placenta	75.4	29	0.7
Repair of current obstetric laceration	75.5–75.6	350	8.8
Manual exploration of uterine cavity, postpartum	75.7	17	0.4
Other obstetrical procedures	Residual	*2	*0.1
Bilateral destruction or occlusion of fallopian tubes	66.2–66.3	313	7.9
Dilation and curettage of uterus	69.02–69.09	17	0.4
Other procedures	Residual	117	2.9
Incidental appendectomy	47.1	20	0.5
Insertion of indwelling urinary catheter	57.96	10	0.3

*Numbers will not add to total because episiotomies are listed in more than one category
Source: *Vital and Health Statistics, Advancedata* No. 83 Oct. 1982

TABLE 4–7.   Cesarean Delivery Rates by Mother's Ethnicity and Marital Status, 1965 and 1978

	Delivery rate		Change in rate (%)
	1965	1978	
Ethnicity:			
White	4.4	15.6	254.5
Other	3.9	14.6	274.4
Not reported	5.4	13.8	155.6
Marital Status:			
Married	4.6	15.5	237.0
Unmarried	3.0	13.3	312.1
Not reported	4.7	18.1	285.1

Source: *National Hospital Discharge Survey*

FIG. 4–2. Cesarean delivery rates by regions of the country, 1965–1978, National Hospital Discharge Survey.

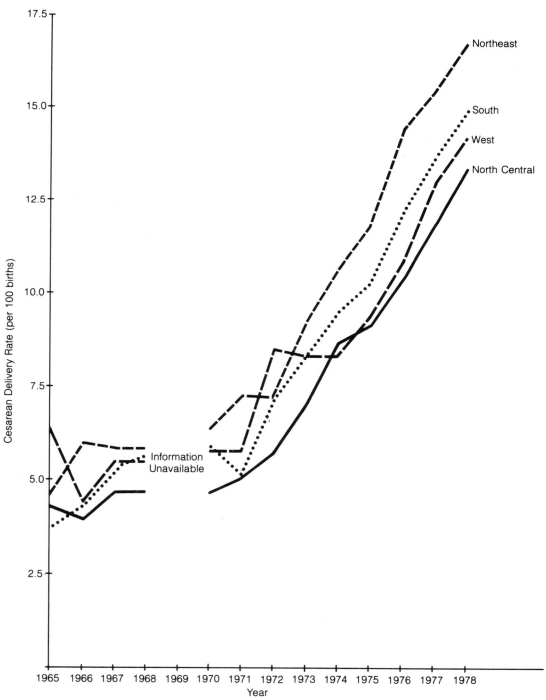

FIG. 4–3.   Percentage of deliveries by cesarean: selected countries, 1970–78.

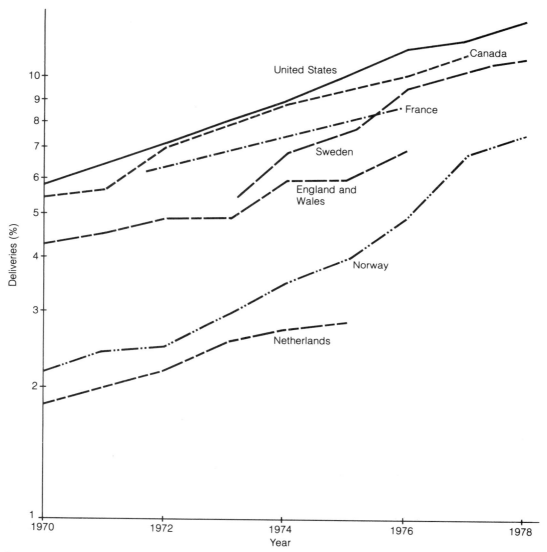

Source: National statistics offices of selected countries, personal communication.

to this phenomenon in the United States. They included increased specialization in obstetrics and increased emphasis on fetal health and survival made possible by technological advances, such as fetal monitoring.

Speculation from more general quarters and from within the medical community itself posits the growing number of malpractice suits against obstetricians and gynecologists as a chief reason for increased cesarean section for problematic deliveries. The diagnoses most closely related to increased use of cesarean delivery between 1970 and 1978 included dystocia (fetopelvic disproportion, abnormal pelvis, prolonged labor), a previous cesarean section, breech presentation, and fetal distress. These four diagnoses accounted for roughly 90% of the increase in cesarean deliveries. Dystocia accounted for 29%, previous cesarean, 27%; breech presentation, 15%, and fetal distress 15%. Another way of looking at the trend is shown in Table 4–8. For example, dystocia was the problem in 6.7% of complicated deliveries in 1978; 67% of women with this complication were delivered by cesarean—up from 50.6% in 1970.

TABLE 4–8. Cesarean Delivery Rate by Complication, and Percentage of All Deliveries Having each Complication, All CPHA Hospitals, 1970 and 1978

COMPLICATION	CESAREAN DELIVERY RATE*		ALL DELIVERIES WITH COMPLICATION (%)	
	1970	1978	1970	1978
No mention	0.2	0.2	69.9	54.4
Lacerations	0.0	0.1	9.8	11.8
Previous cesarean	98.3	98.9	2.1	4.6
Dystocia[†]	50.6	67.0	3.8	6.7
Breech	11.6	60.1	2.9	2.8
Persistent occiput posterior	3.5	10.3	1.4	1.2
Other malpresentations	30.5	37.2	0.8	1.0
Other "maternal"[‡]	38.2	50.5	1.4	1.2
Other "fetal"**	6.3	25.5	2.8	8.0
Other "fetal"—both years[¶]	6.3	14.7	2.8	4.6
Other "fetal"—other‖	NR	40.4	NR	3.4
Other, unspecified	6.1	7.0	5.2	8.3
All	5.7	14.7	100.00	100.00

*Cesarean deliveries per 100 total deliveries
[†]Fetopelvic disproportion, abnormal pelvis, prolonged labor
[‡]Antepartum hemorrhage, prior gynecologic surgery
**Premature ROM, premature labor, multiple pregnancy, prolonged ROM, prolonged pregnancy, fetal distress, ROM (rupture of membranes)
[¶]Premature ROM, premature labor
‖Includes conditions in ** except for those in [¶].
NR Not reported
Source: NIH Pub. No. 82-2067

Historically, it has been difficult to separate the component of cesarean mortality and morbidity due to the operation itself and the underlying complication that may have led to its use. In the 1800's, the mortality rate for cesarean delivery was 75%, this was due in great part to operative risks. Fig. 4–4 illustrates the overall difference in mortality between cesarean delivered and vaginally delivered mothers from 1970 to 1978.

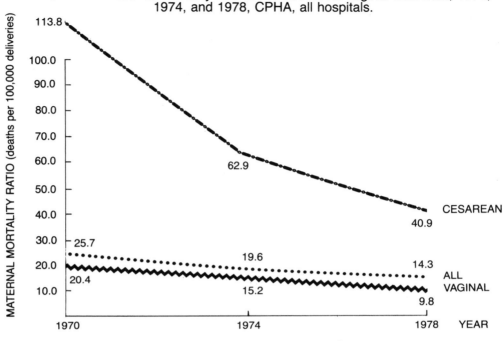

FIG. 4–4.   Maternal mortality ratio for cesarean vs. vaginal deliveries, 1970, 1974, and 1978, CPHA, all hospitals.

Source: NIH PUB. No. 82-2067

Today, cesarean delivery due to a diagnostic indication of previous cesarean has a mortality risk that is just twice as high as that of a vaginal delivery. When done for other diagnostic considerations, the rate is about four times as high.

Cesarean mortality rates in relation to the surgical risks are influenced considerably by the surgeon's skill, the anesthesiologist, and the surgical setting. The greatest operative risks are hemorrhage, infection, and anesthesia.

The task force on cesarean delivery estimated that 15% of direct obstetric maternal deaths resulted from anesthesia, especially from aspiration of gastric contents into the lungs. Endometritis (inflammation of the endometrium), wound infections, and urinary-tract infections are the most common maternal complications from cesarean deliveries.

Cesarean complications are more prevalent than those of vaginal delivery. The higher incidence is due to operative injuries to the urinary tract and bowel, wound abscess, wound rupture, hemorrhage, and paralytic ileus (intestinal obstruction). A comparison of cesarean and vaginal delivery complications is summarized in Table 4–9.

TABLE 4–9. Puerperal Complications, Obstetric Statistical Cooperative, 1973–1977

COMPLICATION	CESAREAN DELIVERY		VAGINAL DELIVERY	
	Number	%	Number	%
Endometritis	3,733	16.11	1,990	1.40
Mastitis	229	1.00	636	2.45
Thrombophlebitis	139	0.60	181	0.13
Infected wound	731	3.16	145	0.10
Peritonitis	114	0.49	16	0.01
Septicemia	91	0.39	26	0.02
Pyelonephritis	1,057	4.56	584	0.41
Urinary retention	102	0.44	3,945	2.78
Oliguria/anuria	19	0.08	24	0.02
Other urinary	504	2.18	771	0.54
Respiratory	438	1.89	306	0.21
Abdominal wound dehiscence	171	0.74	14	0.01
Postspinal syndrome	182	0.79	165	0.12
Psychosis	48	0.21	99	0.07
Other	331	1.43	713	0.50
Total single deliveries	23,169	100.00	142,030	100.00

Source: NIH Pub. No. 82-2067

The controversy over increasing cesarean deliveries and the—sometimes—impersonal atmosphere of hospital delivery have prompted some women to opt for either delivery at home or midwife delivery (Table 4–10). Proponents point to the lower cesarean rate for home deliveries. Critics note that only low risk pregnancies plan to deliver at home or with a midwife.

ABORTION

Teenage fertility data do not reflect the actual number of pregnancies among teenagers. This is because of the increased prevalence of legalized abortion in recent years. Table 4–11 shows the abortion rate for women in each relevant age group, and marital category.

Between 1973 and 1981, the highest abortion rate was for women younger than 15 years—a rate that's mainly rising (Table 4–11). Between 1978 and 1981, the average rate for nonwhite women declined. But the rate for white women continued to rise. Still, the abortion rate for white women is just a little more than one-half that for nonwhite women. Over the entire period between 1973 and 1981, the abortion rate for each age group except that between 30 and 39 years either doubled or more than doubled. Increases in the age groups 30 to 34 and 35 to 39 were considerably less.

The number of reported abortions and their percentage distribution according to pregnancy duration and other parameters is

TABLE 4–10.   Live births by Place of Delivery, Attendant, and Race of Child: United States, 1975–82 (Based on 100% of births in selected states and on a 50% sample of births in all other states)

YEAR AND RACE OF CHILD	Total	IN HOSPITAL*				NONHOSPITAL†			
		Physician	Midwife	Other	Unspecified	Physician	Midwife	Other	Unspecified
All races:									
1982	3,680,537	3,560,644	63,062	11,936	6,554	10,296	14,375	11,855	1,185
1981	3,629,238	3,490,919	55,537	13,303	31,823	10,998	12,754	11,794	2,110
1980	3,612,258	3,499,959	51,576	17,456	7,379	11,992	11,093	11,630	1,173
1979	3,494,398	3,393,773	44,496	11,221	10,994	11,837	10,363	10,032	1,682
1978	3,333,279	3,221,677	36,282	12,721	29,979	11,806	9,778	9,167	1,869
1977	3,326,632	3,203,242	30,635	12,531	47,065	12,766	9,991	7,449	2,953
1976	3,167,788	3,055,287	24,656	12,871	45,282	11,940	9,574	5,914	2,264
1975	3,144,198	3,026,024	19,686	7,122	64,069	11,265	9,727	2,960	3,345
White:									
1982	2,942,054	2,853,427	42,684	8,197	5,116	7,982	13,262	9,982	1,404
1981	2,908,669	2,804,868	37,019	9,405	25,505	8,560	11,577	10,047	1,688
1980	2,898,732	2,815,382	33,730	13,691	5,548	9,495	9,919	10,021	946
1979	2,808,420	2,733,403	29,086	8,380	9,157	9,356	8,879	8,734	1,425
1978	2,681,116	2,598,455	22,319	9,952	23,977	9,136	7,733	8,059	1,485
1977	2,691,070	2,600,011	17,935	9,643	38,056	9,389	7,028	6,605	2,403
1976	2,567,614	2,486,339	13,733	9,642	36,203	8,894	5,824	5,148	1,831
1975	2,551,996	2,465,957	10,076	5,342	52,392	7,818	5,082	2,585	2,744
All other:									
1982	738,483	707,217	20,378	3,739	1,438	2,314	1,113	1,873	411
1981	720,569	686,051	18,518	3,898	6,318	2,438	1,177	1,747	422
1980	713,526	684,577	17,846	3,765	1,831	2,497	1,174	1,609	227
1979	685,978	660,370	15,410	2,841	1,837	2,481	1,484	1,298	257
1978	652,163	623,222	13,963	2,769	6,002	2,670	2,045	1,108	384
1977	635,562	603,231	12,700	2,888	9,009	3,377	2,963	844	550
1976	600,174	568,948	10,923	3,229	9,079	3,046	3,750	766	433
1975	592,202	560,067	9,610	1,780	11,677	3,447	4,645	375	601
Black:									
1982	592,641	568,943	16,162	2,147	1,024	1,868	877	1,364	256
1981	587,797	561,821	15,104	2,113	4,267	1,976	991	1,262	263
1980	589,616	567,568	14,229	2,090	1,321	2,062	1,001	1,170	175
1979	577,855	557,183	13,001	1,856	1,205	2,099	1,356	954	201
1978	551,540	527,861	11,549	1,875	4,906	2,325	1,924	825	275
1977	544,221	518,069	10,295	2,105	6,802	3,044	2,883	578	445
1976	514,479	488,335	8,954	2,480	7,378	2,728	3,675	550	379
1975	511,581	484,416	7,707	1,311	9,595	3,161	4,602	281	508

*Includes births occurring en route to or on arrival at hospital
†Includes births with place of delivery not stated
Source: *Monthly Vital Statistics*. Vol. 33, No. 6, Sept. 1984

shown in Table 4–12. Table 4–13 shows the number of maternal deaths from abortion between 1973 and 1981. From 1973 through 1978, many abortions were performed during the later weeks of gestation—from 16 to 21 or more—raising the maternal death rate in the 13 or more weeks' category. The maternal death rate was highest for these late gestation procedures. By the late 1970s, the rate of abortions performed at 16 to 20 weeks' gestation fell and with it the maternal death rate.

TABLE 4–11. Legal Abortion Ratios,* According to Selected Patient Characteristics: United States, 1973–81 (Data are based on reporting by state health departments and by facilities)

SELECTED CHARACTERIS-TIC	1973	1974	1975	1976	1977	1978	1979	1980	1981
Total	19.6	24.2	27.2	31.2	32.4	34.7	35.8	35.9	35.8
Age (in years):									
Under 15	74.3	92.4	101.5	111.2	112.1	110.2	121.3	122.7	126.4
15–19	31.7	39.9	46.4	54.4	57.2	61.8	66.0	66.4	66.8
20–24	17.9	21.9	25.0	30.1	32.5	35.6	37.3	37.5	37.9
25–29	12.3	15.0	16.6	19.0	19.9	21.6	22.3	23.0	23.2
30–34	16.5	20.5	22.1	23.5	22.8	23.6	23.3	23.3	23.7
35–39	26.7	34.9	37.5	41.1	42.4	43.7	41.5	40.3	40.3
40 and over	40.2	53.8	59.9	68.9	74.2	76.6	74.7	78.3	77.6
Race:									
White	17.5	20.7	22.7	25.6	26.6	28.9	30.7	31.3	31.2
All other	28.9	39.6	46.5	55.1	57.1	58.6	56.8	54.7	54.4
Marital status:									
Married	6.2	7.6	8.3	9.0	9.3	11.0	10.7	10.2	9.8
Unmarried	109.8	132.6	141.1	159.2	158.5	156.7	157.8	149.9	147.5
Number of previous live births†:									
0	23.0	27.4	30.2	35.2	41.1	46.3	48.8	48.6	48.6
1	12.1	15.0	17.3	20.2	19.1	20.8	21.3	21.9	21.9
2	19.6	25.6	29.7	33.0	31.2	32.4	32.7	32.8	32.6
3	25.8	34.6	39.8	44.6	39.3	35.7	34.3	33.5	33.5
4 or more	26.4	35.3	40.8	46.7	41.5	31.6	29.1	27.3	26.6

*Per 100 live births
†For 1973–77, data indicate number of living children
Sources: Centers for Disease Control: *Abortion Surveillance, 1973–78*. Public Health Service, DHHS, Atlanta, Ga., May 1975–Nov. 1980; *Abortion Surveillance, 1979–80*. Public Health Service, DHHS, Atlanta, Ga., May 1983; Unpublished data

TABLE 4–12. Legal Abortions,* According to Selected Characteristics: United States, 1973–81 (Data are based on reporting by state health departments and by facilities)

SELECTED CHARACTERISTIC	1973	1974	1975	1976	1977	1978	1979	1980	1981
Centers for Disease Control	616	763	855	988	1,079	1,158	1,252	1,298	1,301
					Percentage distribution				
Total	100.0	100.0	100.0	100.0	100.0	100.0	100.0	100.0	100.0
Gestation (in weeks):									
Under 9	36.1	42.6	44.6	47.0	51.2	52.2	52.1	51.7	51.2
9–10	29.4	28.7	28.4	28.0	27.2	26.9	27.0	26.2	26.8
11–12	17.9	15.4	14.9	14.4	13.1	12.3	12.5	12.2	12.1
13–15	6.9	5.5	5.0	4.5	3.4	4.0	4.2	5.2	5.2
16–20	8.0	6.5	6.1	5.1	4.3	3.7	3.4	3.9	3.7
21 and over	1.7	1.2	1.0	0.9	0.9	0.9	0.9	0.9	1.0
Procedure:									
Curettage	88.4	89.7	90.9	92.8	93.8	94.6	95.0	95.5	96.1
Intrauterine instillation	10.4	7.8	6.2	6.0	5.4	3.9	3.3	3.1	2.8
Hysterotomy or hysterectomy	0.7	0.6	0.4	0.2	0.2	0.1	0.1	0.1	0.1
Other	0.6	1.9	2.4	0.9	0.7	1.4	1.6	1.3	1.0

SELECTED CHARACTERISTIC	1973	1974	1975	1976	1977	1978	1979	1980	1981
Facility:									
In state of residence	74.8	86.6	89.2	90.0	90.0	89.3	90.0	92.6	92.5
Out-of-state of residence	25.2	13.4	10.8	10.0	10.0	10.7	10.0	7.4	7.5
Previous induced abortions:									
0	. . .	86.8	81.9	79.8	76.8	70.7	68.9	67.6	65.3
1	. . .	11.3	14.9	16.6	18.3	22.1	23.0	23.5	24.3
2	. . .	1.5	2.5	2.7	3.4	5.3	5.9	6.6	7.5
3 or more	. . .	0.4	0.7	0.9	1.5	1.8	2.1	2.3	2.9

*Reported in thousands
Sources: Centers for Disease Control: *Abortion Surveillance, 1979–80*. Public Health Service, DHHS, Atlanta, Ga. May 1983; Unpublished data; Sullivan E, Tietze C, and Dryfoos, J: Legal abortions in the United States, 1975–1976. *Fam. Plann. Perspect.* 9(3):116–129, May–June 1977; Henshaw S, Forrest JD, and Blaine E: Abortion services in the United States, 1981 and 1982. *Fam. Plann. Perspect.* 16(3).

TABLE 4–13.   Legal Abortions, Abortion-related Deaths and Death Rates, and Relative Risk of Death, According to Period of Gestation: United States, 1973–75, 1976–78, and 1979–81
(Data are based primarily on reporting by state health departments and by facilities)

GESTATION AND YEAR	LEGAL ABORTIONS REPORTED	ABORTION-RELATED DEATHS		RELATIVE RISK OF DEATH*
		Number	Rate per 100,000 abortions	
Total:				
1973–75	2,234,160	80	3.6	—
1976–78	3,225,473	37	1.1	—
1979–81	3,850,287	34	0.9	—
Under 9 weeks:				
1973–75	928,814	7	0.8	1.0
1976–78	1,620,840	6	0.4	1.0
1979–81	1,989,506	10	0.5	1.0
9–10 weeks:				
1973–75	642,884	14	2.2	2.8
1976–78	882,051	7	0.8	2.0
1979–81	1,025,656	7	0.7	1.4
11–12 weeks:				
1973–75	355,217	12	3.4	4.2
1976–78	425,744	2	0.5	1.2
1979–81	471,921	6	1.3	2.6
13 or more:				
1973–75	307,245	47	15.3	19.1
1976–78	296,838	22	7.4	18.5
1979–81	363,204	11	3.0	6.0

*The ratio of the death rate in the specified category to the death rate for gestation under 9 weeks
Source: Centers for Disease Control: *Abortion Surveillance, 1978*. Public Health Service, DHHS, Atlanta, Ga., Nov. 1980; unpublished data

Abortions have also changed. Suction curettage has largely replaced dilation and curettage ("D and C") for first trimester abortions. Dilation and evacuation are now performed more often for longer pregnancies, reducing the maternal complication rate and morbidity.

Gynecology 5

Periodic surveys taken by the U.S. government in 1965, 1973, and 1976 provide data on contraceptive use and practice in the decade following the introduction of the birth control pill. The proportion of couples practicing contraception increased from 63.2% in 1965 to 67.7% in 1976 (Table 5–1). Preliminary data from the 1982 survey on family growth indicate a slight decrease in contraceptive practice at 65.6% of all married couples. The decline in the proportion of nonusers between 1965 and 1976 is most striking among those with less than a high school education. This least-educated group, however, still shows the largest percentage of nonusers at 11.2%.

CONTRACEPTION

As might be expected, women married for only a few years use contraceptives less than those married 5 to 9 years or 10 to 14 years. Many of the latter groups have had as many children as they intend to have. In the longest marriages of 15 years or more, contraceptives are used less than in younger marriages this may be explained partly by increased infertility among women older than age 35 years.

TABLE 5–1. Percentage Distribution of Currently Married Women Age 15–44 years, by Contraceptive Status, According to Selected Characteristics: United States, 1965, 1973, and 1976

CHARACTERISTIC	CONTRACEPTIVE STATUS											
	Contraceptors			Pregnancy, post partum, seeking pregnancy			Noncontraceptively sterile			Other nonusers		
	1976	1973	1965	1976	1973	1965	1976	1973	1965	1976	1973	1965
	Percent of currently married women											
Total	67.7	69.6	63.2	13.3	14.3	15.4	11.4	7.5	11.6	7.6	8.7	9.7
Age (in years):												
15–29	68.9	70.2	63.1	22.2	23.0	27.2	3.3	1.3	3.3	5.6	5.5	6.4
15–19	69.4	57.0	55.0	23.6	35.8	36.7	*0.2	*0.4	*0.6	*6.8	6.8	7.7
30–44	66.7	69.1	63.3	5.8	7.0	7.8	18.2	12.6	17.0	9.3	11.3	11.9
Years since first marriage												
0–4	66.9	66.5	57.5	25.4	27.2	35.1	2.0	*0.8	1.7	5.7	5.5	5.7
5–9	70.3	72.7	66.3	20.0	19.2	21.7	4.3	1.7	4.5	5.5	6.4	7.5
10–14	72.5	74.6	68.1	6.6	9.6	11.1	13.3	7.2	11.8	7.5	8.5	9.0
15 or more	64.1	67.3	61.8	2.6	3.2	5.1	22.8	16.8	19.9	10.5	12.8	13.1
Parity and intent to have more children												
All parities:												
Intend no more	70.6	74.7	66.3	4.1	4.6	7.2	17.8	12.1	17.2	7.5	8.6	9.4
Intend more	62.9	60.3	55.6	31.9	33.9	35.6	—	—	—	5.1	5.7	8.8
Parity 0–2:												
Intend no more	68.9	71.8	57.4	6.4	6.9	7.5	16.4	11.3	25.5	8.3	10.0	9.6
Intend more	63.3	60.3	53.6	31.9	34.3	38.3	—	—	—	4.7	5.4	8.1
Parity 3 or more:												
Intend no more	72.6	77.4	72.4	1.6	2.5	6.9	19.3	12.9	11.5	6.5	7.2	9.2
Intend more	54.8	60.8	64.7	31.4	27.6	23.3	—	—	—	13.9	11.6	12.0
Education												
Less than high school	60.1	62.3	56.5	13.7	13.9	15.0	15.0	10.2	13.3	11.2	13.5	15.2
High school	68.0	71.1	65.4	13.5	14.0	15.6	11.5	7.3	12.1	7.1	7.5	6.9
More than high school	73.1	74.4	70.5	12.6	15.1	15.7	8.6	4.8	7.4	5.8	5.7	6.4

*Includes women for whom information on years since first marriage, intent to have more children, or education was missing; also includes women who did not know whether they intended to have more children or disagreed with their husbands about it
Note: Statistics are based on samples of the household population of the conterminous United States
Source: *Vital and Health Statistics*, Series 23, No. 10

Fig 5–1 shows the differential in contraceptive use between black and white women for 1965 to 1976. The proportion of black women using contraceptives increased from 56.2% to 58.6% between 1965 and 1976. Among white women it rose from 64.1% to 68.8%.

A notable increase also occurred among white Catholics. In 1965, 57% used contraceptives. This jumped to 68% by 1976. The increase made the proportion of Catholic users comparable to Protestant users, which was 67% in 1965 and 69% in 1976.

FIG. 5–1.   Percentage of currently married women age 15–44 years, using contraception, by race: United States, 1965, 1973, and 1976.

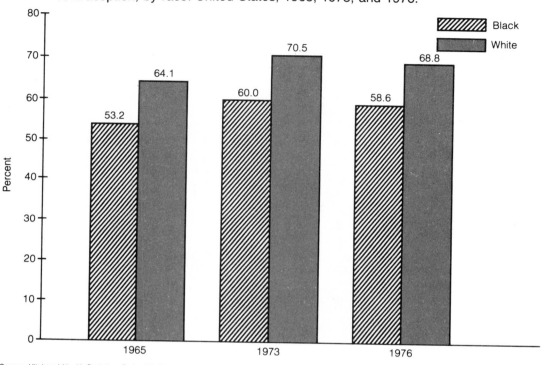

Source: *Vital and Health Statistics,* Series 23, No. 10

According to the 1976 National Survey of Family Growth, those who considered themselves at risk for an unwanted pregnancy reported contraceptive use as: 7.2 million using oral contraceptives; 2.1 million using IUDs; 2.1 million using condoms; 1.0 million using the rhythm method; 0.9 million using foam; 0.8 million using diaphragms; 0.6 million using withdrawal; 0.6 million using other methods.

The choice of contraceptives and corresponding changes over the same decade are shown in Table 5–2. More couples turned to oral contraceptives, the intrauterine device (IUD), and sterilization instead of the traditional methods, such as the condom, diaphragm, foams, or the rhythm method. In 1965, younger women age 15 to 29 years primarily used the pill, whereas older couples age 30 to 44 years used the condom. By 1976, the pill was used by 35.1% of the contraceptors age 15 to 29 years, but sterilization was the leading method of contraception in the older group. Use of condoms by the 30 to 44 years group declined from 44% to 21.9%. Oral contraception reached a peak in 1973 and declined

TABLE 5–2. Percentage Distribution of Currently Married Women Age 15–44 years by Contraceptive Status and Method, According to Age: United States, 1965, 1973, and 1976

	AGE (IN YEARS)								
	15–44			15–29			30–44		
CONTRACEPTIVE STATUS AND METHOD	1976	1973	1965	1976	1973	1965	1976	1973	1965
	Percent distribution								
All women	100.0	100.0	100.0	100.0	100.0	100.0	100.0	100.0	100.0
Contraceptors:									
Total	67.7	69.6	63.2	68.9	70.2	63.1	66.7	69.1	63.3
Sterilization	18.6	16.4	7.8	8.1	7.9	3.9	27.2	23.4	10.4
Nonsurgical methods	49.2	53.2	55.4	60.8	62.3	59.2	39.5	45.7	52.9
Oral contraceptive	22.5	25.1	15.1	35.1	37.6	26.1	12.0	14.8	8.0
Intrauterine device	6.3	6.7	0.8	7.2	8.4	1.1	5.6	5.2	0.5
Traditional methods	20.4	21.4	39.5	18.4	16.2	32.0	21.9	25.7	44.3
Noncontraceptors:									
Total	32.3	30.4	36.7	31.1	29.8	36.9	33.3	30.9	36.7
Pregnant, post partum, or seeking pregnancy	13.3	14.3	15.4	22.2	23.0	27.2	5.8	7.0	7.8
Noncontraceptively sterile	11.4	7.5	11.6	3.3	1.3	3.3	18.2	12.6	17.0
Other nonusers	7.6	8.7	9.7	5.6	5.5	6.4	9.3	11.3	11.9

Note: Statistics are based on samples of the household population of the conterminous United States
Source: *Vital and Health Statistics*, Series 23, No. 10

thereafter as women particularly black women, rejected the pill and the IUD and resumed some traditional methods. Preliminary data for 1982 indicate that use of the pill has declined in the early 1980s to 22.4% of all married women age 15 to 44 years down from the high of 36.6% in 1973.

The percentage of black contraceptors using the pill rose from 30.9% in 1965 to 63.9% in 1973 and then fell to 56% in 1976 (Fig. 5–2). Use by white women went from 42.4% in 1965 to 52.9% in 1973 to 50.6% in 1976. In 1982 (not shown), only 25.1% of black women and 22.3% of white women were using the pill. The marked increase until 1973 is partly attributed to family planning services, while the decline in contraceptives since 1973 reflects increasing awareness of the side effects of oral contraceptives.

The National Reporting System for Family Planning Services estimated that 4,977,000 women visited organized family planning clinics in the United States one or more times during 1980. Seventy-one percent of the women were white. As in earlier U.S. government surveys, the majority of women, particularly those younger than age 30 years, were using the pill. The IUD was more popular among women over 30. Data from the 1965–1976 government surveys show that less than 1% of married women used

FIG. 5–2. Percent of currently married contraceptors 15–29 years of age using the oral contraceptive pill, by race: United States, 1965, 1973, and 1976.

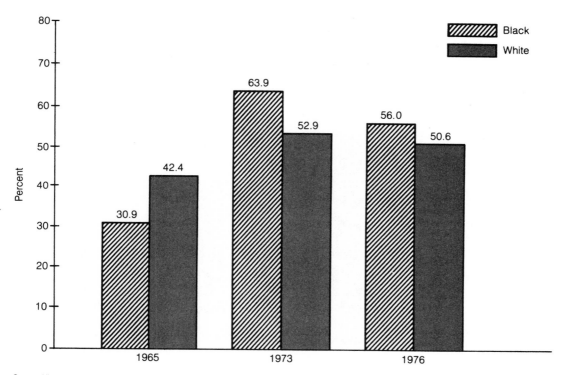

Source: *Vital and Health Statistics*, Series 23, No. 10

IUDs in 1965. This figure rose to about 6% in the 1970s. The 1982 governmental survey on family growth found IUD use at a 10% level in 1976, which fell to 7.9% in 1982. The Copper 7 was the most popular type IUD among women who had not had a child, but the Lippes' loop was the most popular among women who had had two or more children. Health hazards from the Dalkon Shield led to its recall from the marketplace before the release of the data in Fig. 5–3. Since then, other reports about health hazards of the Copper 7 IUD have been published. In 1986 this product was voluntarily withdrawn from the marketplace.

The mortality associated with various methods of contraception has been estimated by the government and various researchers, including Vessey, who studied the incidence of death related to oral contraceptives. These estimates are projected in government Public Health Reports as an annual number for 1981 (Table 5–3).

FIG. 5–3. Percentage distribution of currently married women 15–44 years of age using the IUD at survey date, by type of IUD used: United States, 1976.

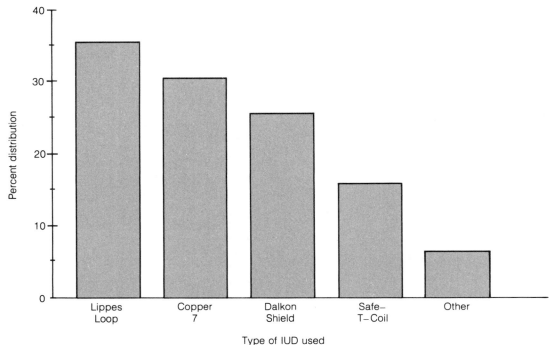

Source: *Vital and Health Statistics Advancedata,* No. 82, June 1980

TABLE 5–3. Deaths Associated with Fertility Regulation U.S. by Age Groups

AGE GROUP (YEARS)	PILL[†]	IUD[†]	TRADI-TIONAL	ABORTION Legal*	ABORTION Illegal*	STERILIZA-TION[‡]	TO-TAL
15–19	33	0	0	2	4	9	48
20–24	105	4	0	11	6	9	135
25–29	72	6	0	3	5	42	128
30–34	248	4	0	4	3	43	302
35–39	132	2	0	2	1	42	179
40–44	190	1	0	4	2	42	239
Total	780	17**	0	25	21	187	1,031

*Source: Centers for Disease Control Abortion Surveillance Branch
[†]Based on Kahn H.S. and Tyler C.W. Mortality associated with use of IUDs JAMA 234: 57–59 Oct 5, 1975: Monthly Vital Statistics Report, Vol 25 No. 7 Supplement Oct 4, 1975. Table 4 Inman W.H.W. and Vessey M.P.: investigation of deaths from pulmonary coronary and cerebral thrombosis in woman of child-bearing age Br Med J (1953). Markush, R.E. and Seigal, D.G.: Oral contraceptives and mortality trends from thromboembolism in the United States. Am J Pub. Health 39, 413–434 March 1969
[‡]Source: Ory H.W. and Greenspan, J. Center for Disease Control Jan 14, 1977 provisional estimates.
**13 of these were using the Dalkon Shield, an IUD no longer used in the United States.

The chance of dying is much higher among smokers who use oral contraceptives than among nonsmokers who use oral contraceptives (Table 5–4).

TABLE 5–4. Mortality Associated with Pregnancy and Childbirth, Legal Abortion, Oral Contraceptives (by smoking status), and IUDs, by Age Groups

| AGE GROUP (YEARS) | PREGNANCY AND CHILDBIRTH* | LEGAL ABORTION† | ORAL CONTRACEPTIVES‡ | | IUDS |
			Nonsmokers**	Smokers**	
15–19	11.1	1.2	1.2	1.4	0.8
20–24	10.0	1.2	1.2	1.4	0.8
25–29	12.5	1.4	1.2	1.4	1.0
30–34	24.9	1.4	1.8	10.4	1.0
35–39	44.0	1.8	3.9	12.8	1.4
40–44	71.4	1.8	6.6	58.4	1.4

*Ratio per 100,000 live births (excluding abortion), United States, 1972–74.
†Ratio per 100,000 first-trimester abortions, United States, 1972–74.
‡Rate per 100,000 users per year.
**Estimates by A.E. Jain.
Source: Tietze, C.: New estimates of mortality associated with fertility control. Fam Plann Perspect 9: 74–76, March-April 1977, Table 1.

STERILIZATION

A correlation is seen between dissemination of information about the dangers of oral contraceptives, especially among smokers and older women, and increased use of sterilization, particularly among older couples. In 1982, 26.6% of ever-married women using some contraceptive were sterilized, as were 13.1% of all married males. The trend toward sterilization among couples married for differing intervals is summarized in Table 5–5.

The trend toward greater use of sterilization, particularly vasectomy, among older couples is not as marked for blacks as for whites. There was a difference of 21% to 5% between whites and blacks in 1976 (Fig. 5–4).

Between 1970 and 1978, tubal sterilization became the most prevalent method of female contraception. About 4.5 million women underwent this procedure in U.S. hospitals. By 1980, the estimated number rose to 5,526,000. Procedures performed yearly increased from 200,000 in 1970 to 700,000 in 1977, the peak year for tubal sterilization.

In 1979 and 1980, the performance rates for tubal sterilization declined slightly to 12.7 and 12.4 per 1,000 women, respectively. The decline, however, may not be real, since currently this procedure is also performed at newly established freestanding ambulatory surgical-care facilities. A 1980 survey estimates that 16,500 tubal sterilizations were performed in such facilities nationwide.

TABLE 5–5.   Percentage Distribution of Currently Married Women Age 15–44 Years Using Contraception by Race and Method of Contraception, According to Years Since First Marriage: United States, 1965, 1973, and 1976

| RACE AND CONTRACEPTIVE METHOD | YEARS SINCE FIRST MARRIAGE | | | | | | | | | | | |
| | 0–4 | | | 5–9 | | | 10–14 | | | 15 or more | | |
	1976	1973	1965	1976	1973	1965	1976	1973	1965	1976	1973	1965
All races★	100.0	100.0	100.0	100.0	100.0	100.0	100.0	100.0	100.0	100.0	100.0	100.0
Modern methods	70.1	77.5	50.3	72.2	72.0	42.6	72.4	66.0	34.6	66.9	62.7	30.7
Female sterilization	1.3	2.4	0.1	10.9	9.9	*2.6	19.0	15.9	9.0	24.0	19.8	11.9
Male sterilization	1.3	1.8	0.5	8.6	8.5	4.4	19.8	14.9	5.7	23.2	18.3	7.4
Oral contraceptive pill	58.8	63.3	47.7	40.2	39.4	33.5	22.4	25.2	19.5	13.5	18.8	10.6
Intrauterine device (IUD)	8.6	10.0	*2.0	12.5	14.2	*2.1	11.1	10.0	*0.5	6.3	5.8	*0.8
Traditional methods	29.9	22.5	49.7	27.8	28.0	57.4	27.6	34.0	65.4	33.1	37.3	69.3
Diaphragm	5.6	2.3	5.0	4.3	3.1	9.0	3.7	3.4	9.8	3.5	4.6	12.6
Condom	9.6	10.3	16.9	8.9	11.4	21.2	10.1	15.0	24.4	13.8	16.6	23.3
Foam	5.4	4.3	5.4	4.3	7.2	3.8	4.5	6.0	3.7	3.5	3.4	*1.9
Rhythm	4.2	2.5	8.9	4.7	2.6	10.0	4.8	4.7	12.3	5.8	5.8	11.3
Withdrawal	2.7	1.4	3.6	3.4	1.7	3.6	2.4	1.6	5.2	3.4	3.2	8.0
Douche	0.6	0.3	4.7	0.5	0.4	*3.5	1.1	0.9	5.3	1.5	1.5	5.9
Other	1.8	1.4	5.2	1.7	1.7	6.3	1.1	2.3	4.7	1.4	2.2	6.4
White	100.0	100.0	100.0	100.0	100.0	100.0	100.0	100.0	100.0	100.0	100.0	100.0
Modern methods	69.9	76.9	52.3	72.5	71.0	42.6	72.5	65.5	33.8	67.3	61.8	29.7
Female sterilization	*1.1	2.2	—	11.0	9.2	*2.1	19.1	15.5	7.7	23.2	18.1	10.8
Male sterilization	*1.4	2.0	*0.5	9.3	8.9	4.7	20.8	15.7	6.2	24.2	19.3	7.7
Oral contraceptive pill	58.8	62.9	50.3	40.0	38.9	33.9	21.3	24.5	19.5	13.7	18.9	10.5
Intrauterine device (IUD)	8.5	9.9	*1.5	12.1	14.1	*1.9	11.2	9.8	*0.4	6.2	5.5	*0.8
Traditional methods	30.1	23.1	47.7	27.5	29.0	57.4	27.5	34.5	66.2	32.7	38.2	70.3
Black	100.0	100.0	100.0	100.0	100.0	100.0	100.0	100.0	100.0	100.0	100.0	100.0
Modern methods	73.0	86.8	37.3	73.9	89.5	38.8	75.2	69.6	43.0	64.9	75.9	42.0
Female sterilization	*4.1	*4.4	*0.7	*11.6	21.0	8.5	24.0	20.0	21.5	36.2	46.2	28.7
Male sterilization	—	*0.1	*0.7	*0.5	*1.3	—	1.7	*4.5	—	*9.0	*1.7	*1.3
Oral contraceptive pill	59.9	70.9	29.9	47.8	51.1	26.4	35.6	31.7	19.8	12.0	16.9	12.1
Intrauterine device (IUD)	*9.0	11.3	*6.0	14.0	16.0	*3.9	*13.9	13.3	*1.7	*7.7	11.2	—
Traditional methods	27.0	13.2	62.7	26.1	10.5	61.2	24.8	30.4	57.0	35.1	24.1	58.0

★Includes white, black, and other races
Note: Statistics are based on samples of the household population of the conterminous United States
Source: *Vital and Health Statistics Advancedata* No. 82, June 1982

Tubal sterilization, although more risky than vasectomy, is often preferred because the latter's a less reliable form of birth control. In tubal ligation, the fallopian tubes are tied, destroyed, or blocked to prevent eggs from traveling from the ovum to the womb. Vasectomy involves cutting the vas deferens, the tube that carries sperm from each testis into the urethra. Although the procedure's regarded as reversible, fertility has been restored in only 50% of vas deferens resections.

More black than white women underwent tubal ligation in the early-1970s. But by 1975, the rate for the latter approached the black rate. After 1975, the rate for blacks once again exceeded the white rate. The racial difference may be explained by the higher parity of black women compared to white and the higher rate of vasectomies among white men compared to black. In other words, black women with larger families are more anxious to avoid additional pregnancies, and their husbands are less likely to have a vasectomy.

FIG. 5–4.   Percentage of currently married contraceptors with wife age 30–44 years using male sterilization, by race: United States, 1965, 1973, and 1976.

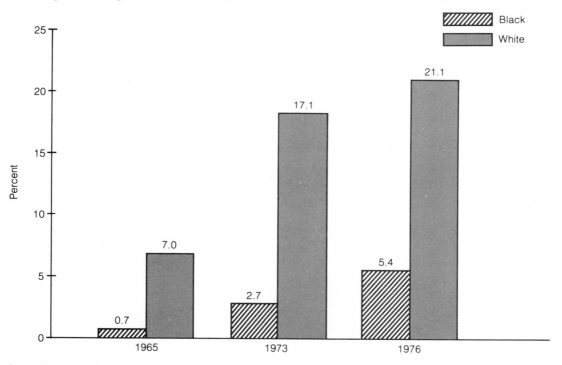

Source: *Vital and Health Statistics*, Series 23. No. 10

Fig. 5–5 shows the rate of tubal sterilization for white women compared to black. Fig 5–6 shows the rate for women by age. The highest rate is for women between ages 25 to 34 years. In 1979 and 1980, the average age for white women was 30 years; for black women, it was 29 years. This is younger than one might expect given the procedure's irreversibility. Efforts to make the procedure reversible continue.

The rate of tubal sterilizations also varies considerably regionally. The highest rate is among southern women, the lowest among western women (Fig. 5–7).

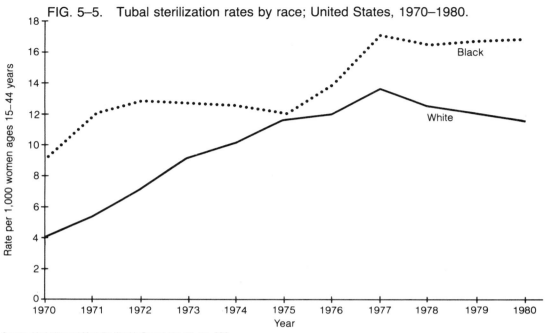

FIG. 5–5.   Tubal sterilization rates by race; United States, 1970–1980.

Source: *Morbidity and Mortality Weekly Report,* Vol. 32, No. 3SS

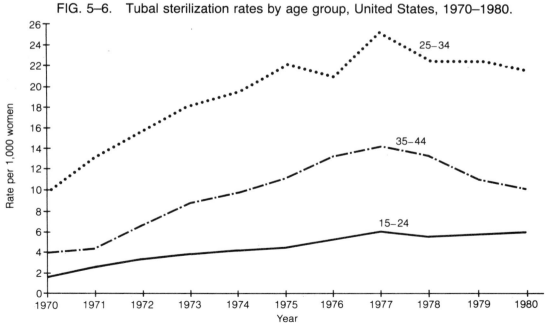

FIG. 5–6.   Tubal sterilization rates by age group, United States, 1970–1980.

Source: *Morbidity and Mortality Weekly Report,* Vol. 32, No. 3SS

FIG. 5–7.   Tubal sterilization rates by geographic region, United States, 1970–1980.

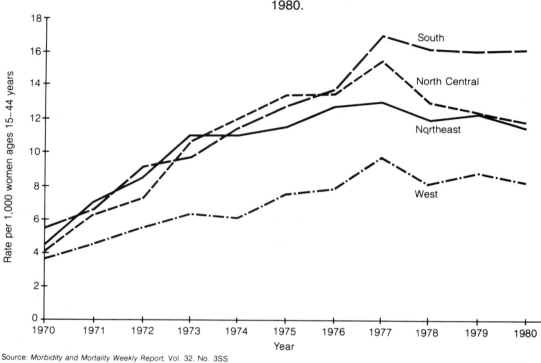

Source: *Morbidity and Mortality Weekly Report,* Vol. 32, No. 3SS

Table 5–6 summarizes the numbers of women who have undergone this procedure for each year between 1970 and 1980 by age, race, and geographic region.

The Centers for Disease Control (CDC) in Atlanta estimate that the in-hospital case : fatality ratio is roughly four deaths per 100,000 tubal sterilizations. Twenty-nine deaths were reported to the CDC between 1970 and 1979. Specific deaths were caused by complications of general anesthesia, sepsis, hemorrhage, myocardial infarction, and others. Three patients whose deaths were sepsis-related had sustained bowel injury following unipolar tubal coagulation. Three of the patients who died from hemorrhage suffered major vessel laceration during laparoscopic sterilization.

HYSTERECTOMY

Hysterectomy is the most common major procedure in the United States and the second most common of all surgical procedures, major and minor. Only dilation and curettage (D and C) is done more often. Between 1970 and 1978, hysterectomies rose by 22% in women between 15 and 44 years old. By the mid-1970s, hysterectomies and D and Cs together represented 10% of all surgical procedures in the United States. Because the trend toward more hysterectomies could ultimately have meant a hysterectomy for one-half of American women government investigators took a harder look at the operation. A congressional and medical panel concluded that as many as 40% of the hysterectomies performed in the mid- and late-1970s may have been unnecessary. A possible consequence of this finding is the decline in the procedure's popularity in recent years.

TABLE 5–6.   Tubal Sterilizations* for Women Ages 15–44 years, by Race, Age, Geographic Region, and Timing in Relation to Pregnancy, United States, 1970–1980

FACTOR	1970	1971	1972	1973	1974	1975	1976	1977	1978	1979	1980
Geographic region:											
Northeast	47	69	89	115	117	124	138	143	131	137	130
North Central	50	75	89	130	148	168	171	200	179	161	158
South	76	90	128	140	169	193	215	270	265	258	279
West	28	34	44	50	51	66	70	89	78	84	84
Age group (years):											
15–24	29	45	60	71	80	83	102	121	112	115	124
25–34	124	172	211	261	290	340	337	413	377	385	395
35–44	48	53	79	102	113	127	154	187	164	141	131
Race:											
White	135	182	236	308	345	412	436	504	472	456	459
Black	45	64	66	67	68	69	84	104	106	109	120
Unspecified	21	23	47	59	71	69	72	93	75	76	72
Timing in relation to pregnancy:											
Not associated with pregnancy	58	98	144	219	266	311	345	396	345	316	307
Pregnancy-associated	143	171	205	216	218	239	247	306	308	324	344
Total	201	269	350	435	484	550	592	702	653	640	650

*Numbers are rounded to the nearest thousand
Source: Data from the National Center For Health Statistics

Reported reasons for a hysterectomy include uterine prolapse, fibroid tumors, cancer, excessive bleeding, or intractable severe pelvic infection. It is also performed prophylactically on patients with precancerous conditions and as a means of sterilization. Sterilization, small fibroid tumors, or uterine polyps are now considered unsound reasons for performing hysterectomies.

In 1978, of women age 40–44 years, 19% had had a hysterectomy. The estimated annual and cumulative prevalence between 1971 and 1978 is shown in Table 5–7.

TABLE 5–7. Hysterectomy: Estimated Annual and Cumulative Prevalence; Rates U.S. Women Ages 15–44, 1971–1978

YEAR (19)	15–19	20–24	25–29	30–34	35–39	40–44	CUMULATIVE RATE: AGES 15–44
1971	0.00	0.12	1.13	3.56	7.93	13.03	3.57
1972	0.01	0.14	1.33	4.07	8.59	13.58	3.78
1973	0.02	0.21	1.58	4.71	9.55	14.34	4.09
1974	0.02	0.25	1.90	5.32	10.44	15.32	4.43
1975	0.02	0.31	2.00	5.80	11.12	16.53	4.71
1976	0.02	0.32	2.21	6.43	11.88	17.54	5.02
1977	0.02	0.34	2.19	6.72	12.37	18.34	5.24
1978	0.03	0.40	2.31	6.89	12.96	19.17	5.52
Relative increase	—	3.3	2.0	1.9	1.6	1.5	1.5

Source: *Morbidity and Mortality Weekly Report Annual Summary*, 1981

If one looks only at the data for simple hysterectomies, namely those that do not involve removal of the ovaries or fallopian tubes (unlike radical hysterectomies or more comprehensive procedures involving hysterectomy in treating advanced pelvic cancer) the cumulative estimate between 1970 and 1980 is 4,342,000. The annual number rose from the 1970 low of 306,000 to 442,000 in 1980 and then fell to 401,000 in 1981. The fall may be due to the rise in tubal ligations in the 1970s as a method of sterilization. The rate in 1979 was 8 per 1,000 women age 15 to 44 years, whereas the rate in 1980 was 7.6.

A histogram of hysterectomies performed in short-stay non-federal hospitals is shown in Fig. 5–8. Since 1975, the rate has been falling, with only one interruption in 1977.

The rate for black women is higher than that for white, although rates for both races have declined. Three-fourths of all procedures nevertheless are performed on white women. Fig. 5–9 shows the rate by race, Fig. 5–10 the rate by age.

Women in the northeast United States had the lowest hysterectomy rate, those in the south had the highest (Fig. 5–11). The higher rate in the south can be partly explained by the greater proportion there of black women, the rate for blacks being higher than the one for whites.

The proportion of vaginal vs. abdominal hysterectomies has also declined in all age groups, races, and regions (Fig. 5–12). While the vaginal hysterectomy involves no abdominal scar, it's more difficult to perform and has a higher rate of postoperative infection.

Those who believe the frequency of hysterectomy is and has been largely justified posit several reasons for its increased use in the early-1970s. The reasons include a possible increase in uterine disease, advances in detecting disease, a desire by women for ster-

FIG. 5–8.   Hospital-performed* hysterectomies performed on women ages 15–44 years, United States, 1970–1980.

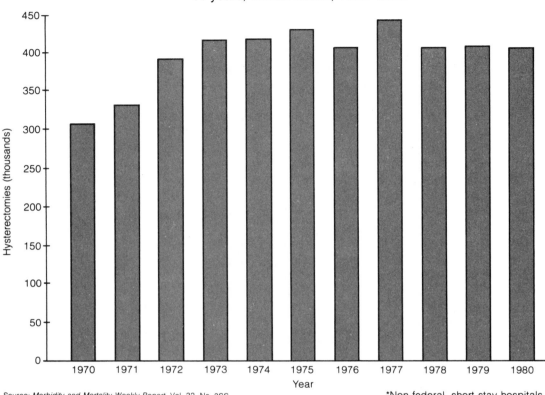

ilization, and increased awareness by women of risks to their reproductive health in the form of early neoplasms, which triggered more frequent checkups.

INFERTILITY

Another contribution to the declining U.S. birth rate is infertility. Of all American couples, 18.5% were voluntarily infertile or contraceptively infertile in 1976. Preliminary data for 1982 show an increased proportion of married couples in this category at 27.8%. Because they do not want to have more children, they are either surgically sterile or practicing contraception. Data from the National Center for Health Statistics in 1976 also indicate that about 6.9 million couples had an involuntary fertility impairment and

FIG. 5–9.   Hysterectomy rates by race, United States, 1970–1980.

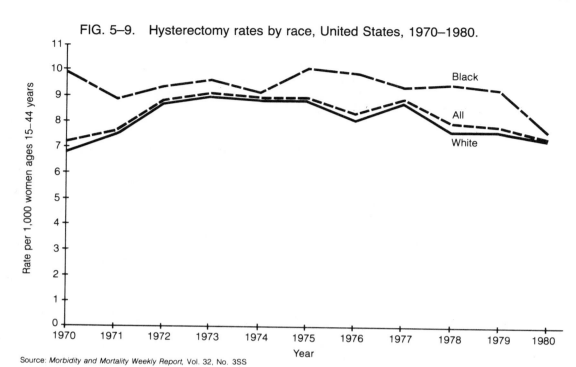

Source: *Morbidity and Mortality Weekly Report,* Vol. 32, No. 3SS

FIG. 5–10.   Hysterectomy rates by age group, United States, 1970–1980.

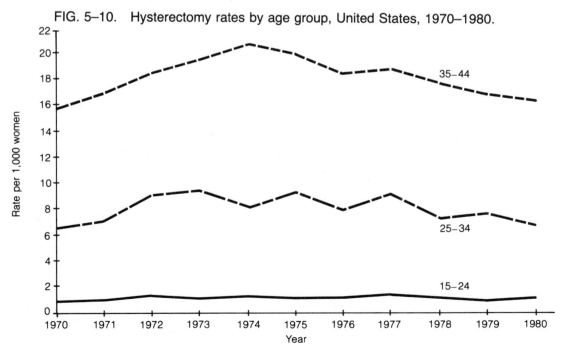

Source: *Morbidity and Mortality Weekly Report,* Vol. 32, No. 3SS

FIG. 5–11.   Hysterectomy rates by geographic region, United States, 1970–1980.

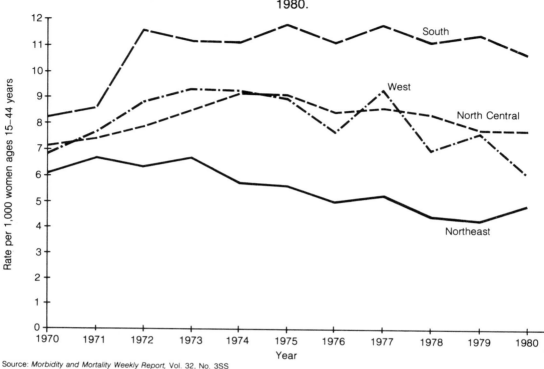

Source: *Morbidity and Mortality Weekly Report,* Vol. 32, No. 3SS

848,000 of them who were childless wanted a baby. In 1982 the number of involuntarily infertile couples dropped to about 6 million, but those who wanted to have a baby rose to 1.4 million. More than 12% of the couples in 1976 who wanted a baby or additional children said that they intended to adopt.

Of the 25.6% involuntarily infertile in 1976, 9.6% comprised couples in which the husband or wife had undergone sterilization for health reasons. But they still wanted more children. By 1982, this proportion constituted 11% of all married couples.

The largest category of the involuntarily infertile was designated "impaired fecundity" in one of the few comprehensive studies of this problem completed by the federal government in the mid-1970s. Several types of couples were classified as having impaired fecundity. The first consisted of couples who were not using any form of contraception who had not had a baby for 3 years of continuous marriage. Theirs was classified as "long interval" impairment; they comprised about 5% of the infertile group. Another subset, the "subfecund" group, consisted of those who responded

FIG. 5–12. Vaginal hysterectomies as a percentage of all hysterectomies for women ages 15–44 years, by race, United States, 1970–1980.

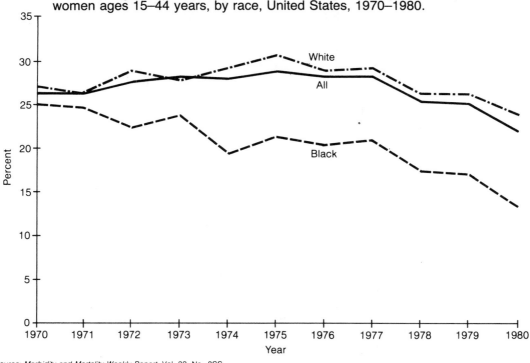

Source: *Morbidity and Mortality Weekly Report,* Vol. 32, No. 3SS

to the study by indicating that they either had difficulty becoming pregnant or maintaining a pregnancy until term. The latter represented about 10.3% of the infertile population. Another 1% were couples who were nonsurgically sterile from accident or illness. Together, these groups comprise 15.7% of involuntarily infertile couples before rounding. But as Table 5–8 indicates, impaired fecundity decreased to 10.5% of married couples in 1982. Many more people had become contraceptively sterile by undergoing surgical sterilization. The percent of voluntarily sterile has increased since 1976. But because of the much larger number of baby boom couples, the number of involuntarily infertile couples has also increased, as mentioned earlier.

Some couples, although in the fecund group, may have an undiscovered fecundity impairment. It may not become apparent until several years of trying to have a baby prove unsuccessful.

Fecundity decreases with age: from 82.1% of all couples when the wife is 20 to 24 years old to 24.3% when the wife is 40 to 44 years old. Some of this decline, however, is the result of voluntary contraception (Table 5–9).

TABLE 5–8. Married Women Age 15–44 years and Percentage Distribution by Fecundity Status, According to Parity and Age: United States, 1976 and 1982 (Statistics are based on samples of the female population of the conterminous United States)

PARITY AND AGE (IN YEARS)	ALL WOMEN		TOTAL		SURGICALLY STERILE				IMPAIRED FECUNDITY		FECUND	
					Contraceptive		Noncontraceptive					
	1982	1976	1982	1976	1982	1976	1982	1976	1982	1976	1982	1976
All parities:	Number in thousands				Percent distribution							
15–44	28,231	27,488	100.0	100.0	27.8	18.5	11.0	9.6	10.5	15.7	50.7	56.1
15–24	4,741	6,020	100.0	100.0	*6.6	3.5	*0.6	*0.4	*8.0	10.8	84.8	85.3
25–34	12,924	12,179	100.0	100.0	23.8	19.1	7.7	6.8	9.4	15.5	59.0	58.7
35–44	10,566	9,288	100.0	100.0	42.3	27.6	19.8	19.4	12.8	19.1	25.1	33.9
Parity 0:												
15–44	5,098	5,235	100.0	100.0	*4.6	1.5	*5.3	4.1	21.7	21.4	68.4	73.0
15–24	1,989	2,738	100.0	100.0	—	*0.2	*0.1	—	*11.1	10.6	88.8	89.3
25–34	2,256	1,931	100.0	100.0	*6.2	*1.8	*3.5	4.5	21.1	27.3	69.2	66.4
35–44	853	565	100.0	100.0	*10.8	*6.5	*22.5	22.3	47.8	53.9	*18.9	17.2
Parity 1 or more:												
15–44	23,133	22,253	100.0	100.0	33.0	22.6	12.3	11.0	8.0	14.3	46.7	52.2
15–24	2,752	3,282	100.0	100.0	*11.3	6.2	*1.0	*0.8	*5.8	11.1	81.9	82.0
25–34	10,668	10,248	100.0	100.0	27.6	22.3	8.6	7.2	7.0	13.2	56.8	57.3
35–44	9,713	8,723	100.0	100.0	45.0	29.0	19.6	19.2	9.7	16.8	25.7	34.9

Source: National Survey of Family Growth

TABLE 5–9. Currently Married Women Age 15–44 years and Percentage Distribution by Infertility Status, According to Age, Parity, and Race: United States, 1965, 1976, and 1982 (Statistics are based on samples of the female population of the conterminous United States)

PARITY, RACE, AND AGE (IN YEARS)	ALL WOMEN (NUMBER IN THOUSANDS):			INFERTILITY STATUS (% DISTRIBUTION):									
					Surgically sterile			Infertile			Fecund		
	1982	1976	1965	Total	1982	1976	1965	1982	1976	1965	1982	1976	1965
Total★	28,231	27,488	26,454	100.0	38.9	28.2	15.8	8.4	10.3	11.2	52.7	61.6	73.0
Age													
15–19	612	1,043	1,032	100.0	0.3	1.0	0.6	2.1	2.1	0.6	97.7	96.6	98.9
20–24	4,130	4,977	4,397	100.0	8.2	4.5	3.1	9.7	6.4	3.5	82.1	89.2	93.4
25–29	6,442	6,443	4,953	100.0	19.6	16.6	9.5	7.0	9.0	6.5	73.4	74.4	84.0
30–34	6,482	5,736	5,074	100.0	43.6	36.2	17.0	7.7	10.3	11.6	48.7	53.5	71.3
35–39	5,783	4,814 }	10,998	100.0	58.2	45.3	22.8	10.2	12.5	14.2	31.6	42.2	63.0
40–44	4,783	4,474 }		100.0	66.7	49.0	26.8	9.0	15.9	20.2	24.3	35.2	52.9
Parity													
0	5,098	5,235	3,492	100.0	9.9	5.6	7.3	19.6	18.1	14.5	70.5	76.3	78.2
1	5,891	5,571	4,497	100.0	17.7	8.8	7.5	10.6	12.4	17.2	71.7	78.8	75.3
2	9,042	7,638	6,878	100.0	46.8	32.3	14.2	5.0	6.0	9.3	48.2	61.7	76.6
3 or more	8,201	9,045	11,587	100.0	63.4	49.8	21.5	3.8	7.9	9.4	32.8	42.3	69.0

PARITY, RACE, AND AGE (IN YEARS)	ALL WOMEN (NUMBER IN THOUSANDS):			INFERTILITY STATUS (% DISTRIBUTION):									
					Surgically sterile			Infertile			Fecund		
	1982	1976	1965	Total	1982	1976	1965	1982	1976	1965	1982	1976	1965
Race and Age:													
White													
15–44	25,175	24,795	23,427	100.0	38.9	29.0	15.9	8.1	9.4	10.5	53.0	61.6	73.6
15–29	10,005	11,217	9,166	100.0	13.7	10.7	5.5	7.4	6.7	4.4	78.8	82.6	90.1
30–44	15,170	13,577	14,261	100.0	55.5	44.1	22.3	8.6	11.6	14.3	35.9	44.3	63.3
Black:													
15–44	2,125	2,169	†3,027	100.0	36.3	21.6	14.2	13.1	18.1	16.3	50.6	60.3	69.5
15–29	859	993	†1,216	100.0	19.7	9.2	6.6	10.9	12.1	4.5	69.4	78.7	88.9
30–44	1,266	1,177	†1,811	100.0	47.5	32.1	20.6	14.6	23.2	26.1	37.9	44.7	53.3

*Includes white, black, and other races.
†Figures are for races other than white.

In 1976, black wives age 15 to 44 years had a larger average number of children than did white ones. Of white couples, 20% had no children, whereas only 11% of all black couples had no children. Of all black couples 24% had had 4 or more children compared with 15% of white couples. Yet there was more subfecund impairment among blacks than whites: 30.2% for blacks with one or more children vs. 24.7% for whites with one or more children. This impairment was embodied in longer intervals between pregnancies in blacks (Fig. 5–13). This relative difference in fecundity remained in 1982 when 13.1% of blacks were infertile compared to 8.1% whites.

The number of spontaneous pregnancy losses in women of different ages is shown in Fig. 5–14. Clearly, the older the woman, the greater the chance of miscarriage.

Infertility is critical today in view of widespread contraception and abortion as well as the willingness of more unwed mothers to keep their babies. Adoption is a difficult option for childless couples. The number of currently married couples with impaired fecundity who wanted a child in 1976 is shown in Fig. 5–15 according to the number of children they already had.

Still, concomitant medical developments may serve as alternatives to adoption. In 1979, a clinic in Norfolk, Virginia began to carry out in vitro fertilization whereby a woman's egg is removed, fertilized in vitro and then implanted in her uterus so that it can be carried to term. This innovative procedure was developed in England and led to the birth of a child there in 1978. The procedure may be a solution to infertility for women with blocked fallopian

FIG.5–13.   Percentage distribution of currently married couples with wife age 15–44 years by fecundity status and race: United States, 1976.

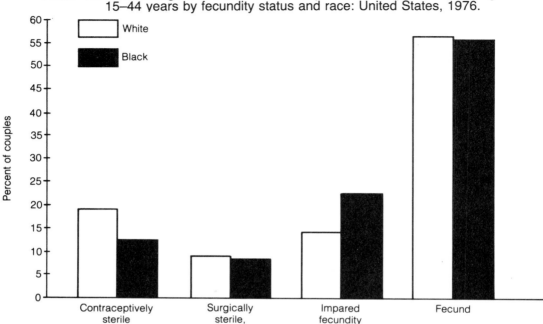

Source: National Survey of Family Growth

FIG. 5–14.   Percentage of currently married women age 15–44 years with one or more reported spontaneous pregnancy losses, by age: United States, 1976.

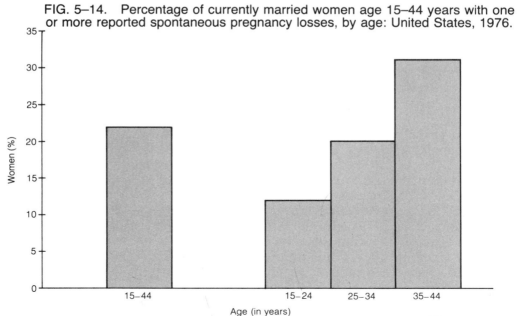

Source: National Survey of Family Growth

FIG. 5–15. Currently married couples with impaired fecundity who want a baby or another baby, by parity: United States, 1976.

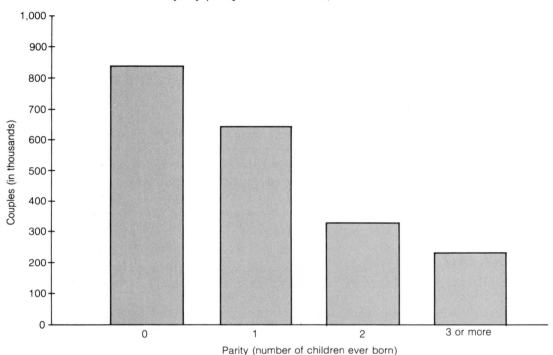

Parity (number of children ever born)

Source: *Morbidity and Mortality Weekly Report*, Vol. 32, No. 3SS

tubes. Since 1981, several infants, so-called test tube babies, have been born in the United States to formerly childless couples.

In other cases of childlessness due to the wife's infertility, a surrogate mother is used. She is impregnated with the husband's semen and carries the baby to term. At birth the child is given to its biological father, and adopted by the father's wife. Such arrangements are usually expensive as well as raising a host of still-unresolved legal and ethical questions.

When a woman is infertile because she doesn't ovulate, she can be treated with several drugs that stimulate the ovaries. Some, such as Pergonal, however, tend to overstimulate the ovaries, causing ovarian cysts or multiple pregnancies.

Infertility is, of course, also a problem in males. When a husband's sperm count is too low to impregnate his wife, the sperm can be collected and in more concentrated form be inserted directly into the wife's uterus. If the husband is fertile but for genetic reasons should not father offspring, the sperm of another donor can be introduced to fertilize the wife's egg in *heterologous insemination*. Although estimates of the number of artificial inseminations (AI) that are performed are unreliable, one that has been offered by medical professionals is that 200,000 people born in the United States over the past 30 years are AI babies. Currently, about 500 physicians perform the procedure; an estimated 8,000 women are artificially inseminated annually.

This practice, although undertaken for several decades in the United States, poses ethical and legal problems, especially when a male donor contributes sperm to a sperm bank. The specimens can then be used to impregnate many women whose children would be related. Conceivably, half-brothers and half-sisters could eventually marry each other or a girl could marry her own father. Offspring have also insisted on meeting their donor fathers, in knowing their medical history, and in some cases, in sharing in their estates.

TOXIC SHOCK SYNDROME

A recently discovered condition indirectly related to the female reproductive system is toxic shock syndrome (TSS), associated with positive cultures for *Staphylococcus aureus* bacteria. Although not exclusively a female complication, TSS primarily develops in young white women using tampons during menstruation. Only 1% of the women were black, with a less than 1% incidence each in hispanic, oriental, and American indian women.

Of 2,204 cases reported to the Atlanta Centers For Disease Control by 1983, 2,108 (96%) were women, 96 cases were men. Of the women, 1,824 were menstruating at onset of TSS; Of those who identified the form of menstrual product they were using during onset, 99% were tampon users. Seventeen cases developed in women using sanitary napkins.

Among nonmenstruating women who developed TSS, infection was reported for a few (4 in 1983) who were using vaginal contraceptive sponges, particularly when the sponge was retained longer than 30 hours without being replaced. A warning now appears on the product packaging urging users to consult their physicians if TSS symptoms develop. Based on reported cases, the risk of death from sponge use does not exceed that associated with other contraceptives ranging from 0.1 to 1.5 per 100,000 women, age 20 to 29 years. The risk of pregnancy-related death is 8.0 per 100,000.

Fig. 5–16 shows the menstruation- and nonmenstruation-related cases of TSS by month from 1979 through 1983.

FIG. 5–16.   Confirmed cases of toxic shock syndrome — United States, 1970–1983.*

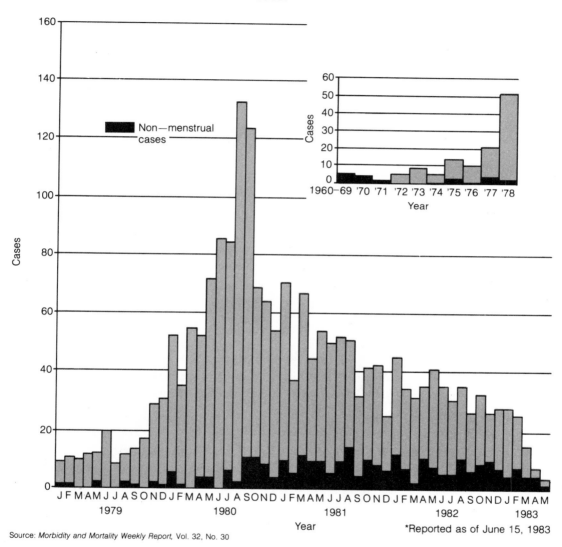

Source: *Morbidity and Mortality Weekly Report,* Vol. 32, No. 30

*Reported as of June 15, 1983

The peak year for reported cases was 1980 (Fig. 5–17). The reported incidence, particularly of menstruation-related cases, is on the decline since 1980. Shifts by states have also occurred since 1980; reported incidence has dropped in California, Wisconsin, and Minnesota. Other states, such as Utah and Colorado, showed an upward spurt in 1982 compared with 1981. Fig. 5–17 shows the 1983 reported cases by state.

FIG. 5–17.   Distribution of definite cases* of toxic shock syndrome, reported by June 15, 1983, United States.

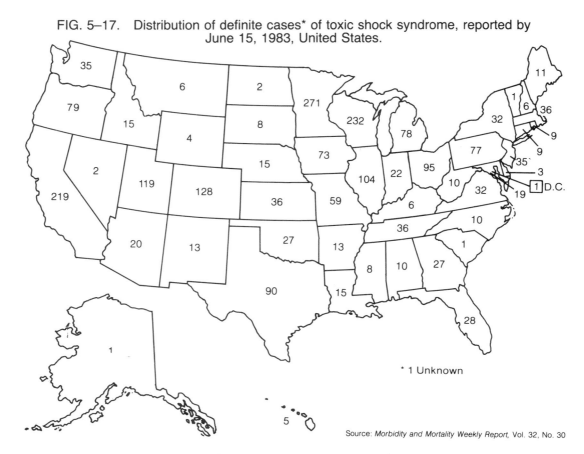

* 1 Unknown

Source: *Morbidity and Mortality Weekly Report,* Vol. 32, No. 30

Symptoms of TSS include fever, hypotension, diffuse rash, nausea, vomiting, and vaginal discharge. Patients are often hospitalized and treated with antimicrobial agents and fluids. Although most patients recover, 103 deaths were reported in the case tally of 2,107, a 5% death rate.

The cases of TSS have triggered removal of Rely tampons from the market and warnings to women about using tampons generally. The decline of the syndrome in the early 1980s and the increased number of nonmenstruation cases being reported reflects the efficacy of these warnings.

DYSMENORRHEA AND PREMENSTRUAL SYNDROME

Primary dysmenorrhea is the sharp, intermittent pain often accompanying menstruation. Unlike secondary dysmenorrhea, which may be due to endometriosis, pelvic inflammatory disease, or tumors, the primary form typically begins just before menstruation and lasts no more than 24 hours. Other menstrual symptoms, which together comprise the premenstrual syndrome (PMS), are nausea; vomiting; headache; diarrhea; abdominal bloating; irritability; and swollen, perhaps painful breasts. On the one hand, at least 10% of all women experience dysmenorrhea pain during menstruation; PMS, on the other, is variable among women and in the same women from month to month.

Although the cause of PMS is still undetermined, some researchers have incriminated premenstrual prostaglandin secretion. Treatment commonly consists of analgesics, such as aspirin, for pain relief. Other therapy involves prostaglandin inhibitors. Oral contraceptives or estrogen are given to suppress ovulation. Patients are occasionally advised to avoid salt as a way of reducing water retention; nutritionists have long recommended calcium supplements to maintain proper fluid-electrolyte balance and to calm disposition; some of them also recommend B-complex vitamins.

ENDOMETRIOSIS

Another painful menstrual condition is endometriosis. Uncommon before age 20, endometriosis usually develops between age 30 and 40 years. Onset can be gradual or sudden, whereas clinical findings become progressively severe until menopause.

The chief symptom is continuous abdominal, pelvic, vaginal, and back pain, beginning the week before menstruation and lasting 2 or 3 days. Extrauterine endometrial tissue, usually around the ovaries in the pelvic area is responsible for the pain. The cause is unknown, but genetic disposition, together with uterine trauma is suspected.

In the early stages, treatment for young women still wanting children may involve androgens. In other patients, progesterone administration eases symptoms by ending menstruation. Surgical treatment, even complete hysterectomy, is often advised for patients in whom endometriosis has become more severe. Infertility occurs in 34% of patients; about 20% of those undergoing gynecologic surgery for other reasons showed advanced endometriosis when examined operatively. In recent years, the incidence seems to be increasing possibly because of delayed childbirth.

MENOPAUSE

The end of menstruation, menopause, occurs in women between age 45 and 55 years. But it can and does occur prematurely in about 5% of women mainly because of ovarian tumors, stress, infection and malnutrition. As menopause begins, women may experience menstrual irregularities or pattern changes, such as spotting, missed or multiple periods during the normal cycle, and changes in the volume and duration of bleeding.

Change in the physical structure of reproductive and other organs can occur, such as reduction in breast size; shrinkage of vulval structures; and loss of subcutaneous fat, pubic hair, and skin elasticity. These changes occur gradually over several years. But women may also develop other signs of menopause, such as irritability, depression, anger, night sweats, vertigo, and palpitations.

One symptom receiving attention today is loss of bone density called osteoporosis. Estrogen replacement therapy prevents osteoporosis and other menopausal discomforts, but not without considerable controversy, since it's incriminated in increased cancer incidence in postmenopausal women. The risk is directly proportional to the length of therapy, multiplying by a factor of 15 in those receiving estrogen supplements for 5 years and doubling in those receiving it for less than 1 year. The advisability of reducing the dosage for those still receiving estrogen has been appreciated by the medical community. Cyclic dosage and progestin supplements have been added to some regimens.

Those clinicians against estrogen replacement therapy state that these measures, especially the cyclic dosage and progestin supplements, do not significantly reduce cancer risk. Patients with a familial history of cancer are not sound candidates for estrogen replacement therapy. Indeed, all treated patients should be monitored regularly. Alternatively, nutritionists advocate daily vitamin-D and calcium supplements for older women. This dietary regimen has long been recognized as a way of preventing bone mineral depletion.

PELVIC INFLAMMATORY DISEASE

Pelvic inflammatory disease (PID) is usually accompanied by lower abdominal pain and a vaginal discharge, with or without low grade fever. It's caused by a bacterial infection in the uterine cavity. So culturing secretions from the endocervix, cul-de-sac, and urethra facilitate antibiotic treatment by identifying the causative pathogen.

Bacteria, such as the causative agents of gonorrhea (*Neisseria gonorrhoeae*) can be introduced through sexual contact. They are a common cause of PID. They can also be introduced by an IUD, abortion, postpartum infection, or pelvic surgery. Other infections of nearby structures, including the appendix and colon, may also precipitate PID.

Often requiring the patient to be hospitalized, the disease can cause sterility or ectopic pregnancy. Treated early, PID can be cured without complication. Occasionally, however, pelvic abscesses rupture. If they do, PID can be life threatening, requiring hysterectomy.

Indeed, PID is the most common serious complication of gonococcal and chlamydial infections; 1 million cases occur annually, leading to 213,000 hospitalizations, 115,000 major pelvic surgeries resulting in permanent sterility, 25,000 ectopic pregnancies, and 900 deaths. The risk of PID is higher in both younger women and the sexually promiscuous. Because younger women are more likely to be promiscuous, they are more often the victims of severe PID, which requires hospitalization. Their higher risk was evident in data from the National Center for Health Statistics Hospital Discharge Surveys conducted from 1975 through 1981. Figure 5–18 shows the age distribution of PID patients.

The hospitalization rate per 1,000 women age 15 to 44 years between 1975 and 1981 according to race, marital status, and geo-

TABLE 5–10.   Pelvic Inflammatory Disease (PID): Rates of Hospitalization, United States, 1975–1981

Factor	Rate*
Race:	
White	4.3
All others	10.6
Marital status:	
Single	4.8
Married	4.9
Divorced	8.4
Separated	7.6
Geographic region:	
Northeast	4.0
North central	5.7
South	6.3
West	4.4
Total PID	5.3

*Per 1,000 women ages 15–44 years
Source: *Morbidity and Mortality Weekly Report Annual Summary* 1983

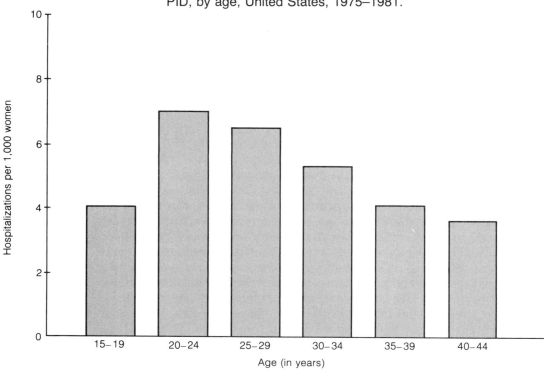

FIG. 5–18.   Pelvic inflammatory disease (PID): Rates of hospitalizations for PID, by age, United States, 1975–1981.

Source: *Morbidity and Mortality Weekly Report, Annual Summary,* 1983

graphic region are listed in Table 5–10. The higher rate of PID for the south correlates with higher rates of venereal disease there. The rising rate of ectopic pregnancies and associated death rate by year for the United States between 1970 and 1980 is shown in Fig. 5–19.

Although a full discussion of veneral disease is beyond the scope of this volume, significant injury to the female reproductive system and to infants born to infected women results directly from an array of veneral infections. Although PID is one of the most common and serious gynecologic complications of venereal disease, especially gonorrhea and chlamydia, it is not dangerous to unborn children. On the other hand, herpes II infections, which are associated with a higher incidence of cervical cancer, can be transmitted to a fetus in utero as well as to an infant as it passes through the birth canal at delivery and can be life threatening. Those infants who survive often suffer severe handicap, including mental retardation.

FIG. 5–19.   Rates of ectopic pregnancies (per 1,000 reported pregnancies) and death-to-case rates (per 1,000 ectopic pregnancies), by year, United States, 1970–1980

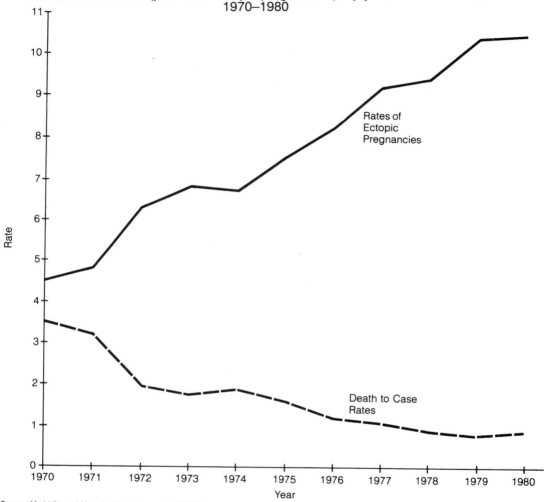

Source: *Morbidity and Mortality Weekly Report,* Vol. 33, No. 2SS

Congenital syphilis in infants younger than age 1 year has been increasing for several years. Obviously, it also poses health risks to the neonate. Thus, buried in the statistics on infertility, maternal and infant injury, handicap and disease is the often-overlooked story of venereal disease. The ever-increasing economic burden running into the billions and the mortality and morbidity caused by venereal disease could be greatly diminished by more responsible sexual behavior.

Pelvic inflammatory disease and toxic shock syndrome, as well as the many other causes of morbidity discussed herein, reflect the great source of jeopardy involved in the natural and everyday process of humankind's self regeneration. It is a challenge for survival that affects those who are healthy and young—infants, children, mothers, and women in their reproductive years. Although the battle for survival is largely being won, the data herein testify to the ongoing struggle of the race to reproduce itself. Needless to say, after overcoming the dangers accompanying the process of regeneration, humankind continues to be threatened by diseases, particularly in advancing age.

A Note On Methodology

This volume and the others in this series are concerned with the demographics of disease, and the disease patterns of different groups of people considered on the basis of age, sex, or cultural grouping. The study of these patterns and the causes of disease in large and small populations is called *epidemiology*.

For thousands of years, people believed that sickness was a punishment for transgressions against the gods. The pattern of sinfulness followed by sickness was evident often enough; for people seldom lived perfect lives and seldom avoided all disease. When sick, they would call for a shaman, a priest-doctor who would beg the gods through prayer and incantation to restore the sick to health.

As simplistic as this approach seems to many modern peoples, the basic impetus of early peoples was epidemiologic. They had isolated a pattern of disease and sought to avoid the scourge of disease by addressing its cause, an angry god.

Gradually, exceptions to the accepted pattern of disease were noticed. Epidemics affected virtually everyone in a community, good or bad. So too, people began to notice other patterns of illness and linked aspects of their natural surroundings, such as their drinking water and certain foods, to the development of disease.

People also noticed that those in contact with a sick person often developed the same symptoms a few days or weeks later.

Thus, a belief developed that disease could be transmitted some-how from person to person, perhaps by the movement of invisible particles traveling from the body of the sick person to that of the well one. The writings of Lucretius described this theory of con-tagious disease. With this pattern of disease noticed, the stage was set for the development of modern epidemiology, the science that looks for the pattern of diseases and the natural causes evidenced by that pattern.

Although the stage was set, many obstacles still had to be over-come. Autopsy examinations were forbidden through most of the Middle Ages, and everyday observational tools used by the modern physician, such as the clinical thermometer and the stethoscope, were not invented until the 17th and 18th centuries, respectively. Thus, it was difficult to diagnose the cause of death in many in-stances. Those who hazarded a guess were often wildly simplistic or incorrect.

Even in the 20th century, influenza, pneumonia, bronchitis and tuberculosis have routinely been mistaken for each other. Autop-sies performed in the latter part of this century finally helped to clarify mortality from these causes.

THE DEATH CERTIFICATE

Despite today's much improved knowledge of the body and dis-ease, the problems of relying on the information entered on a death certificate are notorious. Unfortunately, mortality data reported by countries around the world are based of necessity on death-certificate entries.

In many countries, death-certificate entries represent a physi-cian's diagnosis. But in many other countries, the cause of death is reported by the deceased's relatives to a local clerk. Even in more sophisticated countries, listing the cause of death often ob-scures the real pathologic profile. For example, dying is always a dualistic event resulting from the interaction of a given host and the disease agent that afflicts the host. In one person, influenza may prove fatal because he is constitutionally weak, perhaps from age or other diseases. In another person, encounter with the influ-enza virus would be a minor event—in no way life threatening. But the record of influenza mortality translates simply into the ferocity or danger of influenza as a disease.

The decline in measles mortality throughout much of the 20th century is another example of the confluence of several factors. Until the recent development of the measles vaccine, nothing had changed in the incidence or severity of measles. But mortality in those stricken with pneumonia, a common fatal sequel of measles, was being reduced by sulfur drugs.

Similarly, much information and understanding are lost insofar as death certificates require a listing of only one cause of death, although secondary causes can be listed on the back. Conventions have been established that priority should be given to the cause that is most often fatal, communicable or acute. But such conventions vary from country to country.

This practice becomes increasingly problematic as populations experience greater longevity, since old people often suffer from several conditions by the time they die of any one cited cause. Someone with diabetes, poor renal function, and congestive heart failure (CHF), is taxed by a cold that develops into acute bronchitis. Medication places an added burden on their kidneys. Difficulty in breathing places an extra oxygen demand on their heart, while their blood sugar is difficult to control. After a few days, their kidneys fail as does their heart and they die. Did the cold kill them? Did the bronchitis? Or was the cause of death heart failure, kidney failure, or diabetes? The physician must make a choice. In England and Wales, the death rate from bronchitis is higher than in most other countries. But these UK countries are inclined to list cases like the one described as a bronchitis death whereas other countries tend to list it as a cardiovascular death.

When a death certificate was introduced in England that asked the physician to list death "as consequence of," the number of deaths ascribed to bronchitis doubled. Deaths from nephritis in Canada and the United States doubled as well, while one-third to one-half of the deaths typically attributed to diabetes were counted for some other cause.

DIFFICULTIES OF NOMENCLATURE AND CLASSIFICATION

Beyond these difficulties are ones of nomenclature and classification. To solve these problems, an International Classification of Diseases has been established, which has been revised from time to time. The current code represents the ninth such revision. But in its attempt to standardize diagnosis from country to country, the classification has posed other problems. As knowledge of diseases has increased, the classification has gradually changed from anatomic groupings to etiologic ones. Rheumatic fever is still listed anatomically as a heart disease because it affects the heart. But if it were true to the trend, it would be listed according to cause and would be regarded as an infectious disease because we now know that rheumatic fever is caused by a bacterium and is infectious. In the fourth revision, brain tumors were removed from the category of nervous system diseases and put with neoplasms, as we realized that these tumors are the results of cancerous growth. During the fourth revision of the code, a more mysterious change was the removal of criminal abortion from accidental death to complication of pregnancy.

Over the years, as diagnosis has become more specific, deaths due to ill-defined causes have also decreased and other heretofore ill-defined diseases such as various neoplasms, show increased mortality. As populations have aged and physicians have become accustomed to diagnosing the cause of death in the old, several degenerative diseases, such as diabetes, nephritis, ulcer, and cirrhosis have left the ill-defined category.

CENSUS PROBLEMS

In addition to classification and nomenclature complexities, elementary census biases enter the picture when countries try to calculate their mortality and morbidity rate due to different diseases. These rates are usually expressed as the number of deaths or disease cases per 100,000 population. Sometimes the rates are calculated for men and women separately or for people in different age groups separately. But census numbers are known for their underestimates of population even in advanced countries like the United States. Young children and transient males who travel for their work are often missed in population counts. The 1960 United States census missed an estimated three million people, particularly blacks. Latin Americans tend to report more 5- to 9-year-old children than 0- to 4-year-olds.

Often, information on sex is missing and when asked for their age, people tend to say they are 18 or 21 when these are the ages of majority in a country and 65 when social benefits are available to 65-year-olds. Many people between age 21 and 40 years tend to lower their age when asked. On the other hand, those who do report their true age tend to round their age, especially to even numbers or to ages divisible by five. To compensate for this tendency, researchers often use age intervals when these statistics are compiled.

SURVEYS

Data on morbidity pose yet different problems in that they are usually obtained from health department reports, review of hospital records, or sample surveys of the population. In the United States, physicians are legally obligated to report a large array of diseases, particularly infectious ones, to their health departments. The latter in turn report their data to the Atlanta Centers for Disease Control. Reports come from all of the states, but data gathered independently tend to reveal an under-reporting of disease to the Centers in many instances.

Sometimes hospital records are used for gathering data but these records are often incomplete or have incorrect entries. In addition, hospitalized patients may not reflect the typical patient with a given disease because hospitalized patients are likely to be those who are more severely ill with a specific disease or those who are intractable to less extreme forms of outpatient treatments.

Sample surveys are also subject to misleading findings, depending on how the sample is chosen and how the survey questions are constructed and asked. Data from several large government surveys have been included in this volume. Elaborate statistical sampling methods have been employed to ensure that the surveys are representative. But the questions sometimes fail to elicit pertinent and interesting information. One example can be found in the discussion in Chapter 2 that deals with cerebrovascular disease.

A sample of people were asked about their limitation of normal activity due, presumably, to illness. Some were people who had suffered a stroke; others had not. The stroke victims generally showed greater limitation of activity. But these same people were also generally older and perhaps infirm because of other health conditions. There was no indication that their limitation of activity was specifically related to their stroke event. Thus, we do not know, in light of this particular study, how much dysfunction is caused by stroke in the general population compared to other disability conditions or able-bodied people.

The operations and procedures, together with hospital utilization and physician office visits for people with various diagnoses discussed in this work, were obtained from large government studies, such as the National Ambulatory Care Survey and the National Hospital Discharge Survey, which are conducted annually or periodically. Again the focus of these surveys is not always constant from one to another. Comparison of data from an early survey, such as the NHANES I Nutrition Survey with data on some variables measured by a later survey, such as the NHANES II Survey, is not always possible.

RANDOM VARIABILITY

The perspicacious reader must also realize that health data gathered through survey studies are always subject to a certain amount of random variability. More than a century ago, scientists found to their chagrin that whenever any entity is measured multiple times, the measurement varies. This is true even when the measurement is taken by the same person each time using the same instrument in the same way.

In astronomy, this variability came to be known as the personal equation. But this same kind of variability occurs when one obtains data from a random sample presumably representative of a population of interest. Another random sample surveyed in the same way and equally representative typically yields slightly different results. This variability is called the standard error of a particular study.

The importance of keeping in mind that every sample surveyed has a standard error comes into play when comparisons of data expressed as averages are made. Luckily, the standard error of studies is often small; hence, fairly large differences among groups can be accepted as true differences in reality and not merely the reflection of sampling variability.

When reported differences are small, however, one should not conclude that there is in fact a real difference between two groups unless one knows that the standard error of the study samples is smaller than the small reported difference. For a more detailed explanation of sampling variability see my article, "Randomization and optimal design," *Journal of Chronic Diseases* 36:606–609, 1983.

CRUDE AND AGE-ADJUSTED DATA

Another factor that good health surveys take into account is the age of the groups compared. Clearly, if the blacks interviewed in a study sample were on average 10 years younger than white subjects, one would be mistaken to conclude that whites smoke more than blacks. Obviously, members of groups that smoke to the same degree will show one smoking longer than the other if the members of one group are older than those of the other. The way to correct for age differences when age is likely to affect whether one has an illness or has followed a particular pattern for some time is to compare age-adjusted samples. You will note throughout this volume that crude rates are given as are age-adjusted rates when they are relevant and available.

Since the rates of mortality and morbidity vary among people of different ages, sex, races, and sometimes ethnic and religious backgrounds — particularly in the United States — one has to be mindful of differences in these groups that may account for their differing disease rates. Age is clearly one of these differences that needs to be adjusted for when comparing data. The average and median ages of the black United States population is considerably lower than the white population. Thus, we would expect to see a lower rate of old-age degenerative disease among blacks than among whites when there is no age adjustment. When age is adjusted for or the rate at the same age is compared, epidemiologists have discovered that blacks actually have a higher rate of hypertension than whites.

Another factor not as easily corrected for is access to and utilization of medical resources. If a particular group, such as blacks, are economically less able or socially less inclined to seek medical care when sick, they may ultimately reflect a higher mortality rate from their diseases or a greater morbidity rate as their untreated conditions grow more severe. The higher mortality in such situations should not be regarded as an indication that the higher mortality group has the disease to a greater extent. In other words, blacks may not have more cancer than whites, but they may have a higher cancer mortality rate because they do not receive an early diagnosis or follow treatment regimens for economic or social reasons.

Some researchers speculate that males have a higher general mortality rate than females in part because they tend to seek less medical help for their ailments and fail to follow prescribed treatment regimens for psychological reasons or because it is not convenient for them to see a physician due to career demands.

Aside from the differences in the groups just discussed, differences also exist in groups that may explain why disease does indeed occur more often in some groups than in others. In fact, this is the basic logic of epidemiology and the real incentive for keeping track of vital statistics. Epidemiologists seek to isolate patterns in disease to determine possible pathologic causes.

TELLING PATTERNS

Once it is determined that members of one group are sick and those of another are not, epidemiologists study factors that may be affecting the groups differently. One of the earliest of these investigations was conducted by the physician John Snow who investigated cholera in London between 1848 and 1854. At that time, different parts of London were supplied with water by different companies. Snow noticed that the cholera cases were confined to areas supplied by two specific water companies. In contrast to the others these two obtained their water from a very polluted section of the Thames River.

One of the companies changed its source farther up river and when water pipes were laid in the city, its pipes were alternated with those of the other Thames River company such that each supplied every other house in an area of London that they both served. Snow counted the number of houses in the district served by each company and the number of cholera cases that developed in houses served by each company.

The resulting rates were greatly different, with a much higher rate of cholera in the houses served by the company that was still drawing its water from the polluted source.

This classic study reflects a design referred to as the case control method. This form of research is especially important and useful when one is trying to determine the possible causes of a disease. It has been employed widely and added to our medical knowledge in ways such as the discovery that infant deformities were in the offspring of women who had nothing in common other than ingestion of thalidomide during their pregnancy to the studies that showed a much higher incidence of lung cancer among smokers than among nonsmokers.

Much of the work that has revealed the risk factors for various cancers were obtained from case control studies that compared people with cancer to a group of people without cancer, the control group, which was matched in age, sex, and so on with the disease or case group. Middle-aged women in Aurora, Illinois were reported to have bone cancer more than women in surrounding communities. They seemed like the other women except that they had all worked at a radium dial watch factory in Aurora some years previously, whereas none of the cancer-free control group had worked with the radium. The conclusion was that exposure to radioactive material is a risk factor for developing bone cancer.

Because of modern developments in statistical analysis, researchers also determine possible risk factors when more than one is operative. Such analysis would be used with large cross-sectional community studies that record the prevalence of a disease and other characteristics of the population. The Framingham heart study was of this sort. It revealed that people with heart disease tend to have hypertension, elevated cholesterol readings, and a history of smoking more than those who do not suffer from heart disease.

A follow-up study conducted for several years is currently recording the practices of the offspring of the original study population and the development of heart disease among them. This type of study is called a cohort incidence study because it looks for the development of disease over time. Expensive and lengthy, it is also sometimes impractical.

Each of these designs is useful when one is trying to find the cause of a disease, especially a disease that develops slowly over time. Another type of design that is useful to determine the best form of treatment for a disease is the clinical trial. Some professionals erroneously regard this design as more scientific than the others because the investigator has some control over the exposure of the test sample to a given factor, a treatment of some sort, but this view is incorrect. The randomized controlled trial is subject to many of the same biases as the other designs that I discuss in my article, "The case control or retrospective study in Retrospect," *Journal of Clinical Pharmacology* 21:269–274, July 1981. The debate is moot, however, because the clinical trial cannot be used to determine the cause of a disease. No one can ethically subject healthy people to a factor suspected of causing a disease.

An early example of a clinical trial that *did* test various treatments and also determined the cause of a disease was an investigation made by James Lind into the treatment of scurvy among English sailors in 1747. Sailors long away at sea were afflicted with debilitating scurvy because fresh fruits and vegetables were not storable aboard ship for long periods, and they lacked vitamin C when they went on long voyages.

Lind, on board the *Salisbury*, gathered sailors who were suffering from scurvy and divided them into several groups matched for severity and other factors. He then required that one group take 25 gutts of elixir vitriol daily, another group 2 spoonfuls of vinegar three times daily, another nutmeg, another oranges and lemons, while another group was allowed only a ration of sea water. Within days, dramatic change for the better occurred only in those eating the oranges and lemons.

Lind concluded that eating citrus fruits was essential to the diet of anyone who wished to avoid scurvy and that the disease was caused by the lack of these same fruits in the diet. The British

Navy adopted the policy of serving its sailors limes and lime juice in 1795.

This experiment led Lind to the cause as well as to the treatment of scurvy, yet he did not choose to cause scurvy in the sailors by withholding citrus fruits from the sailors. They were already sick. In this instance, he felt no compunction about giving one group only sea water, which he regarded tantamount to no treatment, a strategy employed today usually with a group of sick people that constitutes a control group.

Ethical considerations can affect such decisions, and often such experiments avoid having a no-treatment group in favor of having several groups each treated differently but all treated with some accepted treatment. The groups are called comparison groups and provide data on which treatment of several possible ones is the best.

The data in *Cancer* present survival information collected from clinical treatment trials as researchers search for the most effective way to fight this disease. Some patients are given chemotherapy in different ways, some radiation treatments in different doses, others undergo surgery, and some receive all three when there is indication that these modalities in combination offer some success. As noted, survival for victims of a given kind of cancer can vary considerably, depending on the treatment.

Readers mindful of these many considerations and of the strategies used by medical researchers to determine what disease patterns exist and how they reveal possible causes of disease will better evaluate the information in this series. They will also better understand why controversy often rages within the medical community about the causes or treatment of disease. And they will better appreciate the remarkable progress achieved by epidemiologists, medical researchers, treating physicians, and policy makers in increasing average life expectancy and eliminating much pain and suffering from normal human existance.

Glossary

Age-adjusted rate: age adjustment, using the direct method, is the application of the age-specific death rates in a population of interest to a standardized age distribution to eliminate the differences in observed rates resulting from differences in population composition

Aorta: the main trunk artery conducting blood from the heart's lower left chamber, originating at the base of the heart

Arrhythmia: an abnormal rhythm of the heart beat

Athetoid: given to involuntary, slow, writhing movements, occurring after unilateral paralysis

Birth rate: a measure dividing the number of live births in a population in a given period by the resident population at the middle of that period; crude birth rate is the number of live births in a year per 1,000 population at mid-year

Cardiovascular: pertaining to the heart and blood vessels

Cohort: any group of people with a common characteristic or set of characteristics that is studied or followed over time

Cyst: a nontumorous sac or vessel containing fluid and foreign matter

Death rate: a measure that divides the number of deaths in a population in a given period by the resident population at the middle of that period

Discharge: according to the National Health Interview Survey, the completion of any continuous period of stay of 1 night or more in a hospital as an inpatient, excluding the stay of a well newborn infant

Diuretic: a drug that promotes the excretion of urine

Edema: swelling due to abnormally large amounts of fluid in body tissues.

Embolism: the blocking of a blood vessel by a clot or other substance in the bloodstream

Hormone: a substance made and secreted by a gland and carried by the bloodstream to other parts of the body, where it has a specific effect on body functions

Incidence: the number of cases of disease having their onset during a particular interval, often expressed as a rate

Lesion: an abnormality in the structure or function of a tissue or body part

Life expectancy: the average years of life remaining to a person at a particular age based generally on the mortality conditions existing in the time mentioned

Lymph: a nearly colorless fluid that bathes body cells and moves through the lymphatic vessels

Marital status: unmarried includes those who are single (never married), divorced or widowed; married typically includes married and separated couples; abortion surveillance reports of the Atlanta Centers for Disease Control count separated people as unmarried for all states except Rhode Island

Morbidity ratio: an arithmetical relationship between the observed cases of disease in a population of interest compared to the cases expected for that population.

Mortality ratio: the deaths from a specific cause in a unit of population in a specified time, such as a year

Neoplasm: any abnormal formation or growth, usually a malignant tumor

Noninstitutionalized population: the population not residing in correctional institutions, detention homes, and training schools for delinquents, homes for the aged and dependent, homes for neglected children, the mentally or physically handicapped, unwed mothers, psychiatric or tuberculosis patients and chronic disease hospitals; the denominator in rates calculated for the National Center for Health Statistics' National Health Interview Survey, National Health and Nutrition Examination Survey, and National Ambulatory Medical Care Survey.

Nosocomial: pertaining to a hospital or infirmary

Parity: a woman's status with respect to the number of children she has had, e.g., nulliparity, primaparity, secundiparity

Prenatal: before birth

Prolapse: a falling or dropping down of an organ or internal part, such as the uterus or rectum

Prevalence: cases of a disease, infected persons or persons with some other attribute present during a particular interval, often expressed as a rate

Puerperium: confinement following childbirth

Radiation: treatment using high-energy radiation from X-rays

Resident population: the population living in the United States, including armed forces and resident foreigners but excluding diplomats

Risk factor: an attribute of a human population or its environment associated with a greater-than-average incidence of disease

Syndrome: a set of symptoms and signs occurring together

Ultrasound: a diagnostic technique in which pictures are made by bouncing sound waves off organs and other structures

X-rays: high-energy radiation used in high doses to treat cancer or in low doses to diagnose disease

Bibliography

Baird D: Epidemiologic patterns over time. *In*: The epidemiology of prematurity. Baltimore: Urban and Schwarzenberg, pp. 5–15, 1977

Berendes HW: Methods of family planning and the risk of low birthweight. *In* Reed DM, Stanley FJ (eds): *The Epidemiology of Prematurity*. Baltimore: Urban and Schwarzenberg, pp. 281–289, 1977

Bergner L, Susser M: Low birth weight and prenatal nutrition: An interpretative review. *Pediatrics* 46: 946–966, Dec. 1970

Berkov B, Sklar J: Does illegitimacy make a difference? A study of the life chances of illegitimate children in California. *Popul Dev Rev* 2:201–217, June 1976

Bolesta LM: The health status of Alaska's Native aging and aged population. *In* The Indian elder: a forgotten American. National Tribal Chairmen's Association, Washington, D.C., 1978: (*a*) pp. 355–368 (*b*) p. 365

Bradshaw BS, Fonner E: The mortality of Spanish-surnamed persons in Texas: 1969–1971. *In* Bean FD, Frisbie WP (eds): The Demography of Racial and Ethnic Groups, New York: Academic Press, pp. 261–282, 1978

Carr BA, Lee ES: Navajo tribal mortality: a life table analysis of the leading causes of death. *Soc Biol* 24:279–287, 1978

Center for Disease Control: The health consequences of smoking. DHEW Pub. No. (CDC) 78-8357. Public Health Service, Atlanta, Ga. 1976

Chase HC, Nelson FG: Education of mother, medical care and condition of infant. Part 3 of a study of risks, medical care, and infant mortality. *Am J Public Health* 63:27–40, Sept 1973 Supp

Churchill JA, et al.: Birth weight and intelligence. *Obstet Gynecol* 28:425–429, Sept 1966

Cooper R, Steinhauer M, Schatzkin A, et al.: Improved mortality among U.S. blacks, 1968–1978: the role of antiracist struggle. *Int J Health Serv* 11:511–522, 1981

Frisbie WP, Bean FD: Some issues in the demographic study of racial and ethnic populations. *In* Bean FD, Frisbie WP (eds): The Demography of Racial and Ethnic Groups, New York: Academic Press, pp. 1–14, 1978

Gee SC, Lee ES, Forthofer RN: Ethnic differentials in neonatal and postneonatal mortality: a birth cohort analysis by a binary variable multiple regression method. *Soc Biol* 23:317–325, 1976

Gundlach, JH: The epidemiologic transition of American Indian mortality. Presented at the annual meeting of the Southwestern Social Science Association, 1981

Hendricks CH: Delivery patterns and reproductive efficiency among groups of differing socioeconomic status and ethnic origins. *Am J Obstet Gynecol* 97:608–624, Mar 1, 1967

Hendricks CH: Twinning in relation to birth weight, mortality, and congenital anomalies. *Obstet Gynecol* 27:47–53, Jan 1966

Holley WL, et al.: Effect of rapid succession of pregnancy, in *Perinatal Factors Affecting Human Development*. Scientific Publication No. 185. Washington, D.C. Pan American Health Organization, Oct. 1969

Hook EB: Changes in tobacco smoking, and ingestion of alcohol and caffeinated beverages during early pregnancy—are these consequences, in part, of fetoprotective mechanisms diminishing maternal exposure to embryotoxins? *In* Kelly S, Hook EB, Janerich P (eds): *Birth Defects, Risks and Consequences.* New York: Academic Press, 1976

Kane SH: Significance of prenatal care. *Obstet Gynecol* 24:66–72, July 1964

Kitagawa EM, Hauser PM: Differential Mortality in the United States: A Study in Socioeconomic Epidemiology. Cambridge, Mass.: Harvard University Press, 1973

Kunitz SJ, Temkin-Greener H: Changing patterns of mortality and hospitalized morbidity on the Navajo Indian reservation. Department of Preventive Medicine and Community Health, University of Rochester School of Medicine and Dentistry, Rochester, N.Y., 1980

Lechtig A, et al.: Effect of food supplementation during pregnancy on birthweight. *Pediatrics* 56:508–520, Oct 1975

Little RE, Schultz FA, Mandell W: Drinking during pregnancy. *J Stud Alcohol* 37:375–379, 1976

Lubchenco LO, et al.: Sequelae of premature birth. *Am J Dis Child* 106:101–115, July 1963

Mantor KG, Poss SS, Wing S: The black/white mortality crossover: investigation from the perspective of the components of aging. *Gerontologist* 19:291–300, 1979

Markides KS, Barnes D: A methodological note on the relationship between infant mortality and socioeconomic status with evidence from San Antonio, Texas. *Soc Biol* 24:38–44, 1977

Nam CB, Weatherby NL, Okay KA: Causes of death which contribute to the mortality crossover effect. *Soc Biol* 25:306–314, 1978

National Center for Health Statistics: A study of infant mortality from linked records by birth weight, period of gestation, and other variables, United States. *Vital and Health Statistics.* Series 20-No. 12. DHEW Pub. No. (HSM) 72-1055. Health Services and Mental Health Administration, Washington. U.S. Government Printing Office, May 1972

National Center for Health Statistics: Congenital anomalies and birth injuries among live births, United States, 1973-74, by S. Taffel. *Vital and Health Statistics.* Series 21-No. 31. DHEW Pub. No. (PHS) 79-1909. Public Health Service. Washington. U.S. Government Printing Office, Nov. 1978

National Center for Health Statistics: Contraceptive utilization among currently married women 15-44 years of age: United States, 1973. *Monthly Vital Statistics Report.* Vol. 25, No. 7, Suppl. DHEW Pub. No. (HRA) 76-1120. Public Health Service. Washington. U.S. Government Printing Office, Oct 4, 1976

National Center for Health Statistics: Life tables: vital statistics of the United States, 1978. Vol. II, sec. 5. U.S. Government Printing Office, Washington, D.C., 1980; (a) p. 13

National Center for Health Statistics: Prenatal care, United States, 1969-1975, by S. Taffel. *Vital and Health Statistics.* Series 21-No. 33. DHEW Pub. No. (PHS) 78-1911. Public Health Service, Washington. U.S. Government Printing Office, Sept. 1978

National Center for Health Statistics: Selected vital and health statistics in poverty and nonpoverty areas of 19 large cities, United States, 1969–71. *Vital and Health Statistics.* Series 21, No. 26. DHEW Pub. No. (HRA) 76-1904. Health Resources Administration. Washington. U.S. Government Printing Office, Nov. 1975

National Center for Health Statistics: Trends and differentials in births to unmarried women, United States, 1970-76, by S. J. Ventura. *Vital and Health Statistics.* Series 21-No. 36. Public Health Service, DHEW, Hyattsville, Md. In press

National Institutes of Health: The women and their pregnancies. *Collaborative Perinatal Study of the National Institute of Neurological Diseases and Stroke.* DHEW Pub. No. (NIH) 73-379, Public Health Service. Washington, U.S. Government Printing Office, 1972 p. 185

Niswander KR et al.: *The Women and Their Pregnancies.* The Collaborative Perinatal Study of the National Institute of Neurological Diseases and Stroke. DHEW Pub. No. (NIH) 73-379. U.S. Dept. of Health, Education, and Welfare. Washington. U.S. Government Printing Office, 1972

Placek PJ: Type of delivery associated with social and demographic, maternal health, infant health, and health insurance factors: Findings from the 1972 National Natality Survey. Paper presented at the American Statistical Association Meeting, Chicago, Ill., Aug. 15–18, 1977

Placek PJ: Maternal and infant health factors associated with low infant birth weight: findings from 1972 National Natality Survey. *In* Reed DM, Stanley FJ (eds): The Epidemiology of Prematurity. Baltimore. Urban and Schwarzenberg, pp. 197–211, 1977

Placek PJ: Underlying medical conditions, complications of pregnancy, and complications of labor to mothers of legitimate live hospital births in the United States. Paper presented at the Population Association of America meeting, Atlanta, Ga., Apr. 13–15, 1978

Roberts RE: The study of mortality in the Mexican American population. *In* Teller CH, et al. (eds): Cuantos Somos: A Demographic Study of the Mexican American Population. Center for Mexican Studies. University of Texas at Austin, pp. 261–282, 1977

Rosenwaike I: The influence of socioeconomic status on incidence of low birth weight. *HSMHA Health Reports.* 86:641–649, July 1971

Schneider J: Low birth weight infants. *Obstet Gynecol* 31:283–287, Feb 1968

Terris M, Gold E: An epidemiologic study of prematurity. *Am J Obstet Gynecol* 103:371–379, Feb 1969

Tietze C: Legal abortions in the United States: rates and ratios by race and age, 1972–74. *Fam Plann Perspect* 9:12–15, Jan/Feb 1977

Van den Berg BJ, Yerushalmy J: The relationship of the rate of intrauterine growth of infants of low birth weight to mortality, morbidity, and congenital anomalies. *J Pediatr* 69:531–545, Oct 1966

Weiss W, Jackson EC: Maternal factors affecting birth weight. *In* Perinatal Factors Affecting Human Development. Scientific Publication No. 185. Washington, D.C. Pan American Health Organization, Oct 1969

Westphal MC, Joshi GB: The interrelationship of birth weight, length of gestation, and neonatal mortality. *Clin Obstet Gynecol* 7:670–686, Sept 1964

Wiener G, et al.: Correlates of low birth weight. Psychological status at eight to ten years of age. *Pediatr Res* 2:110–118, March 1968

INDEX

DATE DUE
